MALPRACTICE DEFENSE: BREAST CANCER

PROFESSIONAL LIABILITY

Other books in the series

Raymond M. Fish and Melvin E. Ehrhardt, *Malpractice Depositions: Avoiding the Traps*, 0-87489-417-4

Raymond M. Fish and Melvin E. Ehrhardt, *Preventing Emergency Malpractice*, 0-87489-464-6

Jack E. Horsley with John Carlova, *Testifying in Court: A Guide for Physicians*, 0-87489-465-4

Melvin M. Belli, Sr. with John Carlova, *Belli for Your Malpractice Defense*, 2nd Edition, 0-87489-550-2

Raymond M. Fish, Melvin E. Ehrhardt, and Betty Fish, *Malpractice: Managing Your Defense*, 2nd Edition, 0-87489-545-6

MALPRACTICE DEFENSE: BREAST CANCER

Campbell F. Watts, MD

MEDICAL ECONOMICS BOOKS
Oradell, New Jersey 07649

Library of Congress Cataloging-in-Publication Data

Watts, Campbell F. (Campbell Franklin), 1918–
    Malpractice defense: breast cancer / Campbell F. Watts.
        p.   cm.
    Includes bibliographical references.
    ISBN 0-87489-576-6
    1. Breast—Cancer—Treatment—Law and legislation. 2. Physi-
cians—Malpractice. 3. Medical jurisprudence. I. Title.
    [DNLM: 1. Breast Neoplasms—legislation. 2. Malpractice. WP
33.1 W348m]
RC280.B8W37 1990
346.7303'32—dc20
[347.306332]
DNLM/DLC
for Library of Congress   89-13450
                                                                                    CIP

ISBN 0-87489-576-6

Medical Economics Company Inc.
Oradell, New Jersey 07649

Printed in the United States of America

CONTENTS

About the Author   vii
Acknowledgments   ix
Preface   xi
 1. Historical Perspective   1
 2. Biologic Predetermination   3
 3. The Natural History of Breast Cancer   9
 4. Diagnosis of Breast Cancer   15
 5. The Camouflaged Tumor   23
 6. The Interval Tumor   31
 7. Common Sources of Error in Clinical Data   35
 8. Avoid the Early Diagnosis Trap   41
 9. Selecting the Medical Witness for the Defense   43
10. Education of the Jury   45
11. Assembling the Medical Facts for the Defense   69
12. The Doubling Time Defense   85
13. The Sliding Threshold Size Defense   95
14. Dispelling Some Common Myths   99
15. When the Plaintiff Challenges the Validity of Your Medical
    Data   109
16. When the Plaintiff Charges That Earlier Detection Would
    Have Meant Longer Life   119
17. How to Deal with the Medical Witness Who Is Never
    Wrong   129
18. Putting It All Together   133
19. Addendum   151
Appendix: Determination of the Malignant Potential of the
Plaintiff's Breast Cancer   155
Glossary   185
Index   193

ABOUT THE AUTHOR

Dr. Campbell F. Watts is a diplomate of the American Board of Surgery. He obtained his M.D. degree from the University of Iowa College of Medicine and his postgraduate training in general surgery at the Mayo Clinic. He received a M.S. in Surgery at the University of Minnesota. The author was engaged in the private practice of general surgery in Cedar Rapids, Iowa, for 35 years. Over the years he developed a special interest in breast cancer and ultimately a large portion of his practice was limited to diseases of the breast. Throughout his career he was a part-time clinical instructor and lectured in the Cedar Rapids hospitals' education and residency program.

Since retiring in 1985, in addition to authoring this book, he has continued to research and lecture on the biology and natural history of breast cancer. He has been especially interested in the cellular and molecular factors that correlate with the aggressiveness of malignancies of the breast.

ACKNOWLEDGMENTS

I am grateful to the many individuals who helped mold our story into its final form. Eighteen months ago the first draft of the manuscript was read by: Frank Mitvalsky, Cedar Rapids attorney; Curt Haas, Cedar Rapids radiation oncologist; David Elderkin, Cedar Rapids trial attorney; Peter Jochimsen, Professor of Surgery at the University of Iowa College of Medicine; and Fred Stamler, Professor of Pathology (Emeritus) at the University of Iowa College of Medicine. These readers agreed that the story needed to be told, and each offered suggestions and corrections that were incorporated into and improved the manuscript.

Mr. Elderkin not only read and reread the manuscript but, over a period of three months, he submitted four long letters of critique. He taught the author what the defense attorney needed to know, why he/she needed to know it, and how best to present it to him/her. It was his idea to lead the reader by the hand through the process of collecting, evaluating, and presenting the data to the jury. Chapters 8, 9, and 10 are largely based on his suggestions.

Susan Love, M.D., of Faulkner Breast Center, Boston, and Jack E. Horsley, J.D., of Craig and Craig, Matton, Illinois, who reviewed the manuscript at the request of the publisher, both made many useful suggestions that were incorporated into the text. Dean Gesme, a Cedar Rapids medical oncologist, kindly reviewed the completed manuscript and made a number of valuable suggestions. We are indebted to Mercy Hospital librarians Linda Armitrage and Joy Stoker Hadow for collecting our source material, and to Penny Warner and Julie Opdahl for their help in typing the manuscript.

The reader is encouraged to submit suggestions or corrections that might make this book a more effective resource for the defense attorney and his/her medical witness.

Campbell F. Watts, M.D.

PREFACE

This book does not pretend to be a comprehensive textbook nor a report of original research on breast cancer. Rather, as the title implies, it is a compilation of data from the medical literature that tells the true story of the natural history and growth pattern of breast cancer. It is the side of the story that the plaintiff's attorney does not mention and juries seldom hear.

Women are constantly bombarded with statements suggesting that early diagnosis of breast cancer is synonymous with cure. Understandably, when a woman is told she has incurable breast cancer, she often concludes that someone must be at fault. Usually she blames the family physician. Is the doctor always at fault? No, I think not. Frequently the unfortunate outcome is the result of the carcinoma itself, something entirely beyond the physician's control. Therefore, the doctor so accused deserves a strong defense. A good defense requires a thorough understanding of the growth pattern and clinical behavior of breast cancer. In addition, both the defense attorney and his/her medical witness should be familiar with the recent expansion of our knowledge in these areas.

There is no defense for a "late" diagnosis secondary to a lack of diagnostic skill or the failure to employ currently accepted diagnostics modalities, and such a defense is not our intent. This book should, however, furnish the reader with the necessary information to decide if the defendant was indeed the victim of the vagaries of the peculiar growth pattern of breast cancer. If this is the case, the book will help the physician prepare a well-organized, logical, and effective defense.

CAVEAT

I am not, and do not pretend to be, an expert in legal strategy. My comments merely reflect the side of the breast cancer story accepted by the vast majority of physicians. Included are suggestions for the education of the jury and other factors that a physician might consider if he/she were responsible for the defense of an alleged failure to make a timely diagnosis of breast cancer. Defense is free to accept or reject these ideas. Hopefully, a few will be helpful.

Campbell F. Watts, M.D.

MALPRACTICE DEFENSE: BREAST CANCER

1

HISTORICAL PERSPECTIVE

There are several reasons why we should study the history of the treatment of breast cancer. First, it makes it easier to understand the natural history of breast cancer. Second, it will enable defense counsel to more effectively examine the plaintiff's medical witness. For no matter how expert, he/she must admit that his/her concept of the pathophysiology and treatment of breast cancer has been wrong for over 50 years. Finally, he/she must admit that his/her current views are not held by all.

PRIOR TO 1900
Breast cancer was treated by simple excision or partial mastectomy. The cancers were huge and there were no cures.

1890 TO 1900
Sampson Handley[1] and William Halsted[2] taught that cancer of the breast spread by local invasion through the breast and via the lymphatics and tissue planes to the regional lymph nodes, which acted as filters. When the lymph nodes became filled, the cancer spilled over into the perivascular lymphatics (the lymphatics surrounding the blood vessels) and spread through these lymphatic channels to the liver, bones, and lungs. *It was thought that breast cancer seldom, if ever, spread through the blood.* Therefore, all agreed that the combination of

1

early diagnosis and radical removal of the breast, underlying muscles, and axillary lymph nodes should result in cure. Radical mastectomy did succeed in reducing the incidence of local recurrence, but no matter how radical the surgery or how much radiation was administered about 50 percent of the patients continued to die of widespread metastatic breast cancer.

1924 TO 1950

Investigators in Europe and Canada began reporting equivalent survival rates using radiation alone or by simple excision of the breast cancer followed by radiation to the breast. For many years these reports were met with skepticism. Only recently were the reports grudgingly accepted.

1950 TO 1987

The extent of surgery for removal of breast cancer was gradually reduced from the mutilating radical mastectomy to simple excision of the breast cancer and a limited axillary dissection. Radiation was usually administered to the entire breast following the "lumpectomy." To the surprise of many, the survival rate remained unchanged. At the present time simple lumpectomy and a limited axillary dissection with or without postoperative radiation is gradually replacing mastectomy as the treatment of choice for early breast cancer.

CONCLUSION

Clearly, the above data demonstrated that at least 50 percent +/− of women with breast cancer have already developed systemic disease prior to the time of surgery. No matter how radical the local treatment is, it will not eliminate systemic breast cancer.

REFERENCES

1. Sampson H. *Cancer of the Breast and its Operative Treatment.* London, 1907.
2. Halsted WS. The results of radical operations for the cure of carcinoma of the breast. *Ann Surg* 46:July 1907

2

BIOLOGIC PREDETERMINATION

Women (and plaintiffs' attorneys) are constantly bombarded by the news media that regular breast examinations, periodic mammography, and monthly breast self-examinations will result in the early diagnosis and cure of breast cancer. No one tells them about the subset of breast cancers that are rapidly growing and aggressive and often metastasize long before they can be detected by any presently available diagnostic modalities. This is the concept of biologic predetermination with which defense counsel should be thoroughly familiar.

Genes are composed of deoxyribonucleic acid (DNA). Segments of DNA that carry specific instructions telling each cell what to do are called genes. There are millions of genes in each human cell. The exact mechanism by which a cancer arises is complex and poorly understood[1]. However, it is thought that when a mutation occurs or a carcinogen or virus gains entry into the nucleus of a breast cell, it can cause damage to the DNA of one of the cell's genes. If one of the damaged genes happens to be one of the genes controlling cell growth, this could be the first step toward the development of a cancer of the breast.

Normally, the damaged DNA of a gene is repaired immediately by the cell[1]. However, if cell division should occur prior to DNA repair, the abnormal genetic message will be copied and become permanent. All future progeny will receive this altered genetic message. One of the functions of some genes (proto-oncogenes) is to attach phosphate molecules to proteins within the cell[1]. Since many of these proteins are enzymes that carry out numerous vital chemical functions within the cell, the behavior of the cell is drastically altered when the structure of the protein is changed. The three most important behavior changes of the new breast cancer cell are:

1. The cancer cells lose the ability to control cell division. Instead of growth in spurts interspersed by long rest periods, the cells grow more or less continuously until the tumor is successfully removed or the host dies.

2. One of the effects of the abnormal attachment of a phosphate molecule to a protein is that some tumors acquire the ability to secrete powerful enzymes or other factors which enable the cancer to invade and metastasize. Thus, some tumor cells (not all and not all to the same degree) acquire the ability to secrete powerful enzymes and other factors which digest the connective tissue surrounding the tumor cell[1,2]. The tumor cell moves into this space, thus invading the local tissues. When the cancer cells reach a blood vessel, the enzymes are somehow thought to make it easier for the tumor cell to gain entry into the blood stream. When tumor emboli lodge in the capillary of a distant organ, the tumor cells continue to grow, giving rise to micrometastases. *There is evidence that when tumors have this ability to invade and metastasize they do so soon after the tumor develops a blood supply—that is, between the tenth and twentieth doubling times, long before the tumor is large enough to be detected by mammography*[3].

3. Cancer cells are genetically unstable. That is, frequent errors of cell division can and do occur. As a result, cancers which at first were slow growing and slow to metastasize can become quite virulent and aggressive. These mitotic aberrations can occur at any time during the life cycle of the breast cancer. However, most investigators are of the opinion that the growth pattern and metastatic potential of a cancer is usually biologically predetermined long before the tumor can be clinically detected.

CLINICAL EVIDENCE SUPPORTING THE CONCEPT OF BIOLOGIC PREDETERMINATION

Consider the following:

1. Breast cancer has a long natural history. Bloom studied 250 cases of untreated breast cancer[4] and the median life expectancy following the clinical onset of the disease was 2.7 years, the five-year survival rate was 18 percent, and the ten-year survival rate was 4 percent. This suggests that some breast cancers are biologically predetermined to grow quite slowly.

2. Some are of the opinion that breast cancer is never "cured." Brinkley and Haybittle[5] followed 704 patients for 31 years. After 25 years the death rate from breast cancer was still 15 times higher than in the general population. This is further proof that there is a biologically predetermined group of breast cancers that grow slowly and have a long indolent life cycle.

3. "Force of mortality"[6] is a consideration. The survival curves of the untreated breast cancer patients of Bloom[4] and Fox[7] were plotted semilogarithmically to determine the "force of mortality," that is, the percentage of patients dying each year. Analysis of these data suggested that there were two subsets of patients.

    a. Sixty percent of the patients had slow-growing indolent tumors. Only 2.5 percent of the patients died of breast cancer each year. (This explains the long natural history of some breast cancers.)

    b. Forty percent of the patients had aggressive tumors. Twenty-five percent of the patients died each year of breast cancer. These data suggest that ". . . there is a subgroup of patients with aggressive breast cancer who die at an annual rate of 25 percent with or without treatment"[6].

    c. Current data suggest that there may be an intermediate group of tumors in which local and regional control affects the overall survival. Unfortunately, the size of this group is unknown and we have not learned to identify these patients[8].

The above, in my opinion, provides powerful evidence

for the concept of biologic predetermination of breast cancer. My own 35 years of experience in treating breast cancer supports this concept.

EXPERIMENTAL EVIDENCE SUPPORTING THE CONCEPT OF BIOLOGIC PREDETERMINATION

Consider also:

1. The metastatic phenotype (the ability of a cell to invade and metastasize) has been transferred from one cell to another by the transplantation of a discrete fragment of DNA from a cancer cell[9].

2. DNA cellular analysis has been done by flow cytometry[10]. Nuclear DNA of a tumor cell is stained with a fluorescent dye and then examined with a laser beam. Computer analysis of the resultant data reveals the degree of distortion of the chromatin pattern of the DNA of the nuclei of the tumor cells. The degree of distortion of the DNA content of tumor nuclei correlates well with prognosis. Tumors with a greater distortion of their DNA pattern are more aggressive and have a poorer prognosis[10]. Since the degree of alteration of nuclear DNA was established at the moment of inception of the cancer, or later as a result of genetic instability, this finding supports the concept of biologic predetermination.

3. Steroid hormone receptors in a tumor cell are a sign of maturity. Cancers without estrogen and progesterone receptors tend to be more rapidly growing and have a poorer prognosis. The presence or absence of steroid hormone receptors is thought to be biologically predetermined.

4. Slamon and colleagues[11] have reported that the amplification of the oncogene (HER-2/neu) correlates well with the survival rate of breast cancer patients. This is further evidence that inherent changes in the DNA of the cancer play a powerful role in determining the future behavior of breast cancer.

SUMMARY

Thus, the degree and nature of the damage to its genetic structure (DNA) by the carcinogen, mitotic aberration, or other unknown factors determine the following:

1. The rate of growth of the cancer cell.
   a. Slow.
   b. Moderate.
   c. Fast.
2. The ability of the tumor cell to secrete the powerful enzymes or other factors that digest the connective tissue surrounding the tumor cell and enable it to invade and metastasize.
   a. Some cancer cells are unable to secrete these enzymes and do not metastasize.
   b. Some cancer cells produce only small to moderate amounts of these enzymes, and the ability to metastasize is variable.
   c. Some cancer cells produce large amounts of these enzymes and metastasize easily and early.

The jury should understand that the aggressiveness or lack of aggressiveness of a tumor is often determined long before the tumor can be detected and may be the single most important factor in determining whether treatment will have a successful outcome or end in failure.

REFERENCES

1. Rensberger Boyce. *Science* 5(7):28–33, September 1984.
2. Liotta LA. Mechanism of tumor invasion. In *Important Advances in Oncology—1985.* Devita, Hellman, and Rosenberg, eds. JB Lippincott, 1985, 28–41.
3. Fisher ER. Impact of pathology on the biologic, diagnostic, prognostic and therapeutic considerations in breast cancer. *Surg Clin N Am* 64(6):1073–1093, 1984.
4. Bloom HJK, et al. Natural history of untreated breast cancer (1805–1903). *Br Med J* 2:213–221, 1962.
5. Brinkley D and Haybittle JL. Long term survival of women with breast cancer. *The Lancet* 1:1118, 1984.
6. Harris J and Henderson IC. Natural history and staging of breast cancer. In *Breast Diseases.* Harris, Hellman, Henderson, and Kinne, eds. JB Lippincott, 1987, p. 233–258.

7. Fox MS. On the diagnosis and treatment of breast cancer. *J.A.M.A.* 241:489–491, 1979.
8. Hellman, S. Primary tumors of the breast. In *Breast Diseases*. Harris, Hellman, Henderson, and Kinne, eds . JB Lippincott, 1987, p. 354.
9. Schnipper LE, Clinical implications of tumor heterogeneity. *N Eng J Med* 314(22):1423–1431, 1986.
10. Feagler JR and Hapke MR. DNA cellular analysis by flow cytometry. *Tumor Conference Letter*, Clarkson Memorial Hospital, Omaha, Nebraska 4(2):1–5, 1987.
11. Slamon DJ, et al. Human breast cancer correlation of relapse and survival with amplification of the HER-1/neu oncogene. *Science* 235:177–182, 1987.

3

THE NATURAL HISTORY OF BREAST CANCER

A clear understanding of the natural history of breast cancer is essential for the construction of a sound defense. The jurors must comprehend the basic concepts of the growth pattern of breast cancer. If they do not, the physician's defense will be doomed to failure.

The following is brief and, admittedly, an oversimplification of the mechanics of the cell kinetics of breast cancer. Well-established breast cancers contain millions of cancer cells that are nourished by a delicate system of blood vessels. Approximately 5 percent of the cancer cells are situated close to the blood vessels and are adequately supplied with nourishment and oxygen. These cells are very active and are constantly growing and dividing to form new cancer cells. They are collectively referred to as the growth fraction of the tumor. Ninety-five percent of the cancer cells, however, are located too far from the blood vessels to obtain adequate nutrition and, as a result, are inactive and do not replicate and produce new cancer cells. (Other complex factors may be involved.)

Since the time required for a breast cancer cell to divide (cell cycle time) is only about 36 hours, and since 5 percent of the tumor cells are constantly and rapidly multiplying, millions of new cancer cells are created in just a few days. However, all of the new cells do not survive. About 50 percent to 75 percent of the new cancer cells are lost (cell loss factor) secondary to necrosis of clusters of cells, necrosis of single cells, and shedding of cancer cells into the lymph and blood stream. When the total number of new tumor cells minus the cell loss factor results in a doubling of the total number of cancer cells within the tumor, one net cell generation of the tumor is said to have taken place (or one tumor volume doubling has occurred).

It will be easier to understand the natural history of breast cancer if we clearly understand the terms *net cell generation (net cell doubling)* and the clinical doubling time of the diameter of the tumor.

NET CELL GENERATION OR NET CELL DOUBLING TIME

When the total number of cancer cells within the tumor has doubled, one net cell generation has occurred. We use the prefix *net* to remind us that we are talking about *the total new cell production minus the cell loss factor.* Table 3–1 gives us an example.

TABLE 3–1. NET CELL GENERATION

# NET CELL GENERATIONS	TOTAL NUMBER OF CELLS IN THE TUMOR
0	1
1	2
2	4
3	8
4	16
5	32
10	1,000
20	1,000,000
30	1,000,000,000 (one billion)
40	one trillion (The human body contains about 11 trillion cells.) Death results when 10 percent of the body consists of cancer cells (numbers are approximated).

CLINICAL DOUBLING TIME (DIAMETER)

When the diameter of a tumor has doubled, its mass has increased eightfold. An eightfold increase in mass requires three net cell generations. For example: If we start with a tumor containing 1,000 cancer cells, then:

	Net Cell
One net cell doubling	2,000 cancer cells
Two net cell doublings	4,000 cancer cells
Three net cell doublings	8,000 cancer cells or an 8x increase in the mass. The diameter of the tumor will have doubled.

Since the growth fraction, the cell cycle time, the cell loss factor, and the malignant potential of breast cancers vary from tumor to tumor, it is not surprising that all breast cancers are not the same. Indeed, there is a tremendous variation in the growth rate and lethality of breast cancers. The time required for the number of cells in a breast cancer to double its diameter varies from nine to over 900 days (average about 100 to 185 days). Thus, while some cancers are indolent and slow growing, others grow rapidly and often metastasize long before they can be detected by any presently available diagnostic modality[1]. These rapidly growing cancers (the interval tumors and the biologically predetermined aggressive cancers) are frequently the basis for malpractice suits[2]. Physicians must learn to identify this subset of breast cancers.

Breast cancer is thought to arise from one cell. At first, the newly formed cancer exists as a small cluster of cells in the extracellular space[3,4]. It contains no blood vessels or lymphatics and derives its nutrients by osmosis from the surrounding extracellular fluid. Cells on the surface of the tumor have an abundant supply of nutrients and, thus, survive and replicate. Cells in the center may die. Since the tumor has no blood supply or lymphatics, shedding of tumor cells into the blood and lymph does not occur.

Judah Folkman and Bert Valle of Harvard[5] have shown that each tumor cell secretes an infinitesimal amount of a chemical called angiogenin. The angiogenin from each tumor cell diffuses into the surrounding tissues for a distance of one to three millimeters, but the amount from one or a few cells has no biologic effect; however, when thousands of tumor cells clustered together each secrete angiogenin, the chemical stimulates the surrounding blood capillaries to grow into the tumor. At first, the new capillaries are quite "leaky" and the tumor cells can easily gain access to the blood stream through gaps in the capillary walls[3–6].

Vascularization of the tumor occurs when the cancer is about 0.3 millimeters in diameter[7].

The 0.3 Millimeter Breast Cancer[7]
Size: one-fourth the size of the head of the common pin.
Age: About three to four years.
Number of doublings: 13 to 14.
Number of cells: 4,000 to 16,000
Comment: Has developed a blood supply. Cancer cells can now shed into the blood. Metastasis can and does occur.

Experimental studies with animal models[6] suggest that as many as 3 to 4 million tumor cells may be shed by a tumor into the blood in a 24-hour period from each gram of tumor tissue. This phenomenon of shedding persists and increases as the tumor continues to grow and becomes better vascularized. Clinical data[8,9,10] confirm the above experimental studies since many operable breast cancer patients have tumor cells in their blood and bone marrow at the time of surgery. Although millions of tumor cells are shed into the blood each day, the vast majority of the shed cells do not survive. Nevertheless, some cells must survive since many authorities are convinced that 50 percent of women already have systemic disease by the time their cancer has reached a diameter of one centimeter[1].

When a tumor has grown to a diameter of two millimeters it will occasionally be visible in a mammogram. The vast majority, however, will not be visible until they have reached a diameter of five millimeters or more.

The Two Millimeter Breast Cancer[7]
Size: Approximately two times the size of the head of a common pin.

Age: About six to seven years.
Number of doublings: About 22.
Number of cells: About 4,000,000.
Comment: Occasionally will be visible in the mammogram. Unfortunately, the vast majority will not be detected by mammography until five to ten millimeters in diameter. Some will never be visible by mammography (see chapter 5). Has been shedding tumor cells into the blood for about three to four years.

A breast cancer is seldom clinically palpable until it reaches a diameter of one centimeter (ten millimeters) unless it is situated on the surface of the breast of a woman with little subcutaneous fat.

The One Centimeter (10 mm) Breast Cancer
Size: About one and a half times the diameter of the eraser on an ordinary lead pencil.
Age: About nine years.
Number of doublings: About 30.
Number of cells: About 1 billion.
Comment: Has been shedding cancer into the blood for about five years, and 50 percent of women have developed systemic disease. It is biologically an old tumor since it has completed three-quarters of its life cycle (30 doublings). Forty doublings usually result in the death of the host.

Many breasts are quite dense and difficult to examine, and the average breast cancer will grow to a diameter of two to four centimeters in diameter before it is detected by the patient or her physician. In one large National Surgical Adjuvant Breast Project study, the average size of the breast cancer at the time of diagnosis was 3.4 centimeters[1].

The 3.4 Centimeter Breast Cancer
Size: Almost one and a half inches in diameter.
Age: About 11 to 12 years.
Number of doublings: About 33.
Number of cells: About 3 to 4 billion.
Comment: Has been shedding cancer cells into the blood for approximately six to seven years.

The Large Breast Cancer (5 cm³)
Size: Massive and systemic.

Age: About 12 to 13 years.
Number of doublings: About 40.
Number of cells: About 1 trillion.
Comment: Usually results in death of the host.

REFERENCES

1. Fisher ER. The impact of pathology on the biologic, diagnostic, prognostic, and therapeutic considerations in breast cancer. *Surg Clin N Am* 64(6):1073–1093, 1984.
2. Spratt JS, et al. Acute carcinoma of the breast. *S.G.O.* 157:220–222, September 1983.
3. Gimbone MA and Gullino PM. Neovascularization induced by intraocular xenografts, normal, preneoplastic, and neoplastic mouse tissues. *J Nat Cancer Institute* 56:305–318, 1976.
4. Brem S, et al. Prolonged tumor dormacy by prevention of neovascularization in the vitreous. *Cancer Research* 36:2807–2812, 1976.
5. Folkman J. Angiogenesis and its inhibitors. In *Important Advances in Oncology—1985.* Devita, Hellman, and Rosenberg, eds. JB Lippincott, 1985, pp. 42–62.
6. Butler P and Gullino PM. Quantitation of cell shedding into efferent blood of mammary adenocarcinoma. *Cancer Research* 35:512–516, 1975.
7. Spratt JS and Spratt JA. Growth rates and the cytokinetic behavior of breast cancer. Lecture presented at the University of Heidelberg, October 1986. Personal communication.
8. Watne A, et al. The prognostic value of tumor cells in the blood. *Arch Surg* 82:48–53, 1961.
9. Engell HC. Cancer cells in circulating blood: clinical study on occurrence of cancer cells in peripheral blood and in venous blood draining tumor area at operation. *Act Chir Scand Supp* 201:1–70, 1955.
10. Redding WH. Detection of micrometastases in patients with primary breast cancer. *The Lancet,* December 3, 1983, pp. 1271–1274.

4

DIAGNOSIS OF BREAST CANCER

THE TRUTH ABOUT EARLY DIAGNOSIS

For many years surgeons were taught that if only surgery for breast cancer were more radical and more meticulous, survival rates would improve. This was false. Millions of frightened women were mutilated by the unnecessary and cruel radical mastectomy. Now, we are told that early diagnosis will cure more than 80 percent of breast cancers. This statement has not been proven. It is true that many studies during the past 10 to 20 years have reported increasing survival rates for breast cancer. However, most thoughtful investigators conclude that these increased survival figures are illusory and secondary to:

1. Changes in the methods of measurement of survival rates.

2. Lead time bias which refers to the diagnosis of breast cancer patients with systemic disease at an earlier stage of the life cycle of the cancer. The resultant increase in the time period from diagnosis to recurrence or death for many patients gives the illusion of an increase in the survival rate. The total survival rate, however, remains unchanged.

3. Overdiagnosis bias. McKinnon[1] stated, ''. . . progressively greater efforts to diagnose and treat cancer early has caused a progressively greater intake of borderline lesions, many of low or no lethal potentiality.'' The increasing popularity of screening mammography has increased the significance

15

of selection bias which falsely improves the survival rates. During the last 20 years, the use of mammography has almost asymptotically increased in usage with no survival advantage thus far[2]. There has been no improvement in the age-adjusted mortality rate as reported by the U.S. Bureau of the Census and the U.S. National Center for Health Statistics.

NO IMPROVEMENT IN THE SURVIVAL RATE

In 1952 McKinnon[1], an epidemiologist from the University of Toronto, stated, "It is disappointing, if not shocking, to find that neither in any province of Canada nor in Massachusetts nor in Wales nor in England has there been any decline in recorded breast cancer mortality [in the last 25 to 30 years]."

In the August 10, 1985, issue of *Lancet* Petr Skrabanek[3] stated that most, if not all, of the survival improvements reported for breast cancer were secondary to lead time bias. The survival rate has not been improved; rather, the survival clock was started sooner.

In the June 1987 issue of *Scientific American*[4] the United States General Accounting Office study was said to have concluded that between 1950 and 1982 there had been no significant improvement in the survival rate of breast cancer. Any reported survival improvements were said to be secondary to measurement changes.

In May 1986, Bailer and Smith[5] reported that they could find no evidence of reduction of the age-adjusted mortality from breast cancer during the years 1950 to 1982. They found no evidence that the vigorous efforts to screen for breast cancer have had an effect on survivorship. Any reported impact was said to be secondary to a staging shift. I agree with Bailer and Smith[5] and McKinnon[1] in the conclusion that any mortality reduction for breast cancer should be reflected in changes in trends and differences between trends of cancer mortality as shown in vital statistics. Thus far, screening programs for breast cancer have produced no such changes.

For a screening program to be effective, it must be possible to diagnose the cancer before metastases have occurred. Therefore, we must determine:

1. At what size can the cancer first be detected by conven-

tional methods (the so-called threshold size)?

2. At what size does the breast cancer first metastasize (the so-called critical size)?

3. What is the time interval between the threshold size and the critical size (the cancer control window)?

The Threshold Size

The threshold size[6] is the size at which the tumor is first detectable. Most radiologists have difficulty detecting invasive breast cancers until they reach a diameter of 2.1 millimeters to five millimeters. However, in some women with dense breasts containing certain types of tumors it may be impossible to visualize these lesions in a mammogram, or even palpate them, until they reach a diameter of one centimeter, two centimeters, or even larger. Thus, the threshold size of the breast cancer may vary from 2.1 millimeters to two or even three centimeters $+/-$.

The Critical Size

The critical size[6] is the size of the cancer at which metastasis first occurs. This point is difficult to determine. Although the precise time cannot be established, there is considerable evidence that metastasis (when it does occur) frequently does so before the breast cancer reaches a diameter of one centimeter[7–11].

1. Bauer[10] estimated that 90 percent of breast cancers have metastasized by the time the tumor reaches a diameter of six millimeters.

2. Donegan[12] stated that the Ellis Fishel State Cancer Hospital data contained seven breast cancers with a diameter of less than one centimeter. Three of these (42 percent) developed distant metastases.

3. Frankl[13] found that 20 percent of occult cancers of the breast found only by mammography had metastasized to the axilla. It is estimated that if these patients harbored microscopic foci of systemic breast cancer it would require about ten years for these lesions to become demonstrable.

4. Pickren[14,15] found a breast cancer eight millimeters in diameter with metastasis to 11 axillary nodes.

5. Biologic predetermination may be a factor. Many investigators are of the opinion that when a tumor contains cells capable of invasion and metastasis they will do so within the first 10 to 20 doublings of the tumor[7] long before these lesions can be detected by any known method. In other words, from the moment of its inception or early in its life cycle, as a result of mutation, most tumor cells either have or do not have the ability to secrete the powerful enzymes and other factors that enable it to invade and metastasize. If the tumor cells have this capability, they will invade the local tissues and, when the tumor becomes vascularized (between the tenth and twentieth doubling), the cancer cells will penetrate the wall of a blood capillary and spread systemically via the blood stream[7,11,16].

CONTRARY OPINION

No one disputes that many breast cancers develop distant metastases long before the tumor can be detected clinically. However, there is disagreement regarding the probability of remote metastases relative to the size of the tumor. As we have said repeatedly, many authors are of the opinion that 50 percent or more of breast cancers have spread systemically by the time the tumor has reached a diameter of one centimeter. Others consider these estimates are too high; see table 4–1 for examples.

These retrospective investigations are subject to all of the biases inherent in such studies.

Summary

There is much evidence that the time interval between the moment a cancer becomes clinically detectable and the time it metastasizes may be a negative value for many patients or, if

---

TABLE 4–1. SYSTEMIC SPREAD OF BREAST CANCERS BY TUMOR SIZE

SIZE OF TUMOR	REFERENCE	% PATIENTS WITH REMOTE METASTASES
1.0 cm.	Koscielny et al. [17]	27% (approximated)
2.8 cm.	Berg & Roggin [18]	50%
3.5 cm.	Koscielny et al. [17]	50%

it is a positive value, the interval may be short. This would explain why no one can demonstrate that delay in diagnosis of one to nine months results in a decrease in survival. The true value of screening programs and early diagnosis will remain in doubt until it can be demonstrated that they have resulted in a decrease in the age-adjusted breast cancer mortality rates as shown in vital statistics. This is the only method that will eliminate lead time bias and selection bias.

DELAY IN DIAGNOSIS AND SURVIVAL RATE

A search of the literature regarding the effect of a delay in diagnosis on the survival rate of breast cancer yields conflicting reports. Many authorities have found little or no difference between the duration of symptoms and the survival rate of breast carcinoma. Others report a definite decrease in the survival rate of breast cancer following a delay in diagnosis. How can we explain this discrepancy? Almost all of the reported studies have been retrospective in nature. It is well known that retrospective studies are seriously flawed by a number of biases such as lead time, length, selection, and so on. (see chapter 7 for a discussion of these biases.) As yet, no retrospective study has been devised that will eliminate these biases. They can only be eliminated by a large, well-run, controlled, prospective, and randomized study. One such study was conducted by the National Surgical Adjuvant Breast Project and reported by E. Fisher and associates[8]. In this study, the duration of symptoms (delay in diagnosis) and the survival rates of 1,665 patients with breast cancer were compared. The patients were classified according to the duration of symptoms: zero to one month, one to three months, three to nine months, and nine-plus months. This study failed to disclose any consistent relationship between the duration of symptoms and the survival in patients with breast cancer. *The authors concluded that the fact that delay in diagnosis did not decrease survival might be secondary to the relatively early metastases of breast cancers.* They stated, ''It would appear from our data that even prompt treatment such as within a month does not universally improve prognosis.''

Spratt[19] has stated, ''There is powerful correlation between the proliferation rate (the growth rate) of cancer and survivorship. This correlation between growth rate and survivorship is confirmed by the consistent observation that there is no relation between the duration of symptoms and survivorship." For example:

Correlation Growth Rate and Survivorship

Duration of Symptoms:	The cancers often are:
Lengthy	Slowly growing/good prognosis.
Brief	Rapidly growing/poor prognosis

The truth is sometimes painful. The fact remains, however, that most thoughtful investigators readily admit that biologic predetermination and that intangible factor of host resistance often have more influence on the survival rate of breast cancer than does early diagnosis[20]. In the meantime, of course, early diagnosis should still be our goal since sometime in the future (unfortunately not at the present time) patients with a low tumor burden of micrometastases may be cured with effective chemotherapy and immunotherapy. Nevertheless, the statement that "early diagnosis always means cure" is a gross oversimplification of the problem and, thus far, has not been proved[20].

CAVEAT

We are not attempting to defend a "late" or missed diagnosis secondary to a lack of diagnostic skill or failure to employ currently accepted diagnostic procedures. We are, however, suggesting that the unfortunate outcome of many breast cancers is secondary to the biology of the breast cancer rather than physician error.

REFERENCES

1. McKinnon NE. Cancer mortality. The failure of control through case finding programs. *S.G.O.* 94:173–178, 1952.
2. Jochimsen P. Personal communication.
3. Skrabanek P. False premises and false promises of breast cancer screening. *The Lancet*, August 10, 1985, pp. 312–320.

4. Editor. Science and the citizen. *Scientific American*: 25, June 1987.

5. Bailer III and Smith M. Progress against cancer. *N Eng J Med* 314:1226–1232, 1986.

6. Heuser L, et al. Relation between mammary cancer growth kinetics and the intervals between screening. *Cancer* 43:857–862, 1979.

7. Fisher ER. The impact of pathology on the biologic, diagnostic, prognostic, and therapeutic considerations in breast cancer. *Surg Clin N Am* 64(6):1073–1093, 1984.

8. Fisher ER, et al. A perspective concerning the relation of durations of symptoms to treatment failure in patients with breast cancer. *Cancer* 40:3160–3167, 1977.

9. Baum M. Primary treatment of operable breast cancer. Reviews on endocrine related cancer. *Cancer* 13:15–18, 1983 (Supplement).

10. Bauer WC, et al. Quoted by Skrabanek, P. False premises and false promises of breast cancer screening. *The Lancet*, August 10, 1985, p. 316.

11. Schabel FM. Concepts for systemic treatment of micrometastases. *Cancer* 35:14–24, 1975.

12. Donegan WL. Quoted by Heuser L. *Cancer* 43:857–862, 1979.

13. Frankl G. Xeromammography and 1200 breast cancers. *Radiologic Clinics of North America* 21(1):81–89, 1983.

14. Pickren JW. Personal communication with Heuser L. *Cancer* 43:857–862, 1979.

15. Pickren JW. Significance of occult metastases. *Cancer* 14:1266–1273, 1961.

16. Liotta LA. Mechanisms of tumor invasion. In *Important Advances in Oncology—1985*. Devita, Hellman, and Rosenberg, eds. JB Lippincott, 1985, pp. 28–41.

17. Koscielny K, Tubiana M, et al. Breast cancer: relationship between the size of the primary tumor and the probability of metastatic dissemination. *Br J Cancer* 49:709–715, 1984.

18. Berg JW and Robbins GF. Factors influencing short and long term survival of breast cancer patients. *S.G.O.*

122:1311, 1966 (data modified by Koscielny[17]).

19. Spratt JS and Spratt JA. Growth rates and the cytokinetic behavior of breast cancer. Lecture presented at the University of Heidelberg, October 1986. Personal communication.

20. Gullino PM Natural history of breast cancer. *Cancer* 39:2697–2703, 1977.

5

THE CAMOUFLAGED TUMOR

In spite of the superficial location of the breast, under certain circumstances even the most astute clinician may be unable to detect a breast cancer until it is two or three centimeters in diameter or occasionally even larger. Philip Stax[1] has stated, "It is generally agreed that up to 20 percent of cancers may not be apparent to the palpating fingers of even the most expert examiner. . . ." In addition, he stated, "It should be emphasized that neither palpation nor mammography used singly or in combination can detect 100 percent of cancers (of the breast)." In all of the National Surgical Adjuvant Breast Protocols (N.S.A.B.P.)[2] involving breast cancer, there has been a mandated follow-up program designed to detect a cancer in the second breast at an earlier state. The follow-up program consisted of: (1) monthly breast self-examinations, (2) physical examination of the breast every six months by a physician, and (3) mammograms every 12 months. In spite of this meticulous clinical surveillance of the remaining breast, the average size of the second carcinoma was 2.4 centimeters—only one centimeter less than that of the first cancer. "This reaffirms the difficulty in clinically recognizing small or 'early' breast cancers."

THE PROBLEM OF BREAST DENSITY

The glandular structure of the breast is embedded in fibrous connective tissue and fat. If the proportion of fibrous and/or

23

glandular tissue is greater than the proportion of fat, the breast will be dense as in the teenager and young adult. Usually the fat content of the breast increases with age and the breast becomes softer, less dense, and easier to examine both clinically and by mammography.

When the breast becomes severely involved with the overgrowth (hyperplasia) of fibrous connective tissue and/or glandular tissue, as is seen in cystic disease, adenosis, or periductal connective tissue hyperplasia, the breast will have an unusually high proportion of fibrous and glandular tissue as compared to fat. These breasts can be extremely dense and are difficult to examine both clinically and by x-ray.

THE PROBLEM OF BREAST CONSISTENCY

The breast involved with chronic cystic mastitis may not only be dense and rubbery but often is riddled with fluid-filled cysts. These cysts vary in size from microscopic to several centimeters in diameter. The resultant diffuse nodularity of a dense breast makes physical examination of the breast even less accurate.

Overgrowth of fibrous tissue (connective tissue hyperplasia) can occasionally produce diffuse nodularity of the breasts. These nodules are solid, quite firm, and vary in size from several millimeters to two centimeters in diameter. When they are numerous, accurate examination of the breast is exceedingly difficult.

THE PROBLEM OF BREAST SIZE

The large dense breast can easily "hide" a cancer with a diameter of several centimeters from the fingers of the most skillful examiner.

THE PROBLEM OF TUMOR DENSITY

When the average person thinks of cancer, he or she thinks of a tumor consisting of nothing but cancer cells. This is not the case. Many tumors contain more benign stromal tissue (benign supporting connective tissue framework) than cancer cells. Thus, breast cancers contain varying amounts of benign tissue elements such as[3]:

Benign Tumor Elements Found in Breast Cancer	Comment
Residual benign breast tissue	35 to 79 percent of a breast can-
Fibroblasts	cer may be composed of benign
Myofibroblasts	stroma[8]
Endothelial cells (blood vessels)	
Granulocytes	
Macrophages	

To look at it another way, the concentration of cancer cells within a breast cancer varies from 21 percent to 65 percent[3]. Obviously, the density of a breast cancer will vary according to the composition of the tumor, especially the proportion of fibrous tissue.

In addition, some tumor cells elaborate soluble factors that diffuse away from the cancer cells and stimulate the fibroblasts and myofibroblasts within the stroma of the tumor and in the tissue surrounding the tumor to proliferate locally and/or se-crete excess matrix components such as fibrous connective tis-sue[4]. When this occurs, the density of the tumor will in-crease. Thus, the density of a breast cancer can at times equal that of the most dense breast. Some tumors are especially prone to mimic the denseness of benign breast tissue[5]: almost all tumors can become camouflaged when the circumstances discussed above exist.

EXAMPLES OF TUMOR CAMOUFLAGING

Some cancers of the breast invade the surrounding tissues in such a manner that the tumor becomes camouflaged from the clinician's examining fingers and at times even from the penetrating rays of the x-ray machine.

1. The Infiltrating Lobular Carcinoma

These tumors frequently present as a "masked" or camou-flaged tumor (47 percent in one series)[6]. They often have a peculiar pattern of invasion which can produce a subtle and vague thickening of the breast without mass formation[7]. Tu-mors with diffuse spreading tumor cells often stimulate the production of little fibrous tissue which tends to be evenly distributed. At times the cancer may produce scattered tiny

25

nodules of cancer which are no larger than a grain of sand. Palpation of the breast sometimes gives the sensation of tiny grains of sand buried deep in the breast tissue[7]. This treacherous tumor often has vague, indistinct borders, and occasionally no overt mass will be apparent until the tumor reaches a diameter of two or three centimeters. Since these tumors seldom form microcalcifications, mammography is of little help until the cancer becomes quite large.

2. The Infiltrating Duct Cell Carcinoma

The common infiltrating duct cell carcinoma also often presents as a camouflaged tumor. (42 percent in one series)[6]. It, too, is dangerous, especially when situated in a dense breast. The density (the firmness or hardness) of this tumor will vary significantly depending on the composition of the tumor. Consider the following:

Fibrous stroma. Many infiltrating duct cell carcinomas stimulate the overgrowth of fibrous connective tissue (desmoplasia) within and around the tumor and, as a result, are quite firm. On the other hand, some tumors fail to stimulate this overgrowth of connective tissue and, as a result, are much less dense. This variation in density enables some of these tumors to match the density of the breast.

Ratio of tumor cells to stroma. When the connective tissue stroma is scanty and the tumor cells are abundant, the tumor will be softer and less dense.

Tumor borders. Although most tumor borders will be stellate, serrated, or circumscribed, a few tumors will have indistinct borders[7]. These tumors may be more difficult to palpate and to visualize by mammography.

Intraductal carcinoma component. This is considered to be a preinvasive carcinoma which is confined to the ducts. However, when it is associated with an invasive breast cancer, some investigators (not all) are of the opinion that it may represent spread of the cancer's cells within the ductal system[7]. The intraductal component does not stimulate the overgrowth of fibrous tissue that is commonly observed in infiltrating duct cell carcinoma. As a result, the intraductal component often is not palpable by the clinician and even the surgeon will have difficulty identifying it at the time of surgery[8]. This pattern of growth can be difficult to detect unless microcalcifications are identifiable by mammography. Many invasive duct cell carcinomas contain no areas of intraductal carcinoma. On the other hand, there are a number of carcinomas that are primarily composed of intraductal carcinoma and have only small areas of infiltrating duct cell carcinoma. These tumors can be difficult to detect by palpation.

How frequently does the infiltrating cell carcinoma contain significant amounts of intraductal carcinoma?

Fisher and associates[9] studied 964 invasive breast cancers. The degree of involvement with intraductal carcinoma varied. In three-fourths of the tumors the intraductal component was considered to be absent or slight. In some tumors, however, the intraductal component was as high as 99 percent. Twenty-eight, or 1 percent, of the tumors contained more than one-third intraductal carcinoma; 11.2 percent contained more than two-thirds intraductal carcinoma. Thus, many infiltrating duct cell carcinomas contain a large proportion of tumor that is difficult, and sometimes even impossible, for the clinician to palpate.

3. The Intraductal Carcinoma

This is a carcinoma situated within the ducts of the breast with no evidence of invasion[4]. Thus it would qualify as a carcinoma-in-situ or a preinvasive carcinoma. When these tumors contain no deposits of calcium within the ducts, they can easily present as a camouflaged tumor (9 percent of the cases in one series)[6].

4. The Medullary Carcinoma

These cellular tumors tend to be well circumscribed[7]. The tumor does not stimulate an overgrowth of connective tissue within or surrounding the tumor (desmoplasia); as a result, these tumors are soft and difficult to palpate. Their smooth circumscribed border enables them to mimic certain benign tumors. These tumors are often two to four times larger than one would expect from the mammogram[10]. When the density of the tumor is similar to that of the breast and the tumor contains

27

no microcalcifications, *it can be impossible to detect by mammography.*

THE PROBLEM OF TUMOR BORDERS

Some breast cancers have sharply circumscribed "pushing-type" borders (about one-third of tumors) and tend to be more easily detected by palpation and mammography. Other tumors are more invasive and tend to have indistinct infiltrative borders which tend to be less dense and more difficult to palpate and more difficult to visualize by mammography.

THE PROBLEM OF TUMOR LOCATION

Tumors situated deep in the breast or against the chest wall may be more difficult to detect.

THE CAMOUFLAGED TUMOR (BY MAMMOGRAPHY)

Since the proportion of the various stromal elements and the concentration of the tumor cells in a breast cancer vary considerably, so will tumor density. It may be impossible to detect a neoplasm by mammography when: (1) the density of the breast and tumor are similar; (2) the cancer contains no calcifications (about one-third contain no calcifications); (3) the cancer produces no secondary changes in the breast, such as skin edema, skin dimpling, etc.; and (4) the cancer does not alter the normal architecture of the breast. Since these tumors are masked or hidden in the mammogram, they have been called the "camouflaged tumor." In addition, the configuration of the breast may not permit certain areas of the breast to be imaged satisfactorily, and these "blind spots" may contain tumors that will not be seen in the mammogram.

In my own experience, approximately one-tenth to one-fifteenth of breast cancers will qualify as camouflaged tumors by mammography.

THE CAMOUFLAGED TUMOR (BY PALPATION)

Rarely, a cancer situated on the surface of the breast may be detected by palpation when it is only three to five millimeters in diameter. Normally, however, a diameter of one centimeter is considered to be the threshold size for the detection by palpation of an "early" breast cancer. There are many situations when the threshold size may be much larger. The threshold size will be larger when: (1) the breast is very dense; (2) the breast has a density similar to that of the tumor; and (3) the tumor is located in the mid-breast or deep breast, especially if the breast is normal in size or is large.

Under these circumstances the threshold size (palpation) will be much larger than a diameter of one centimeter. I have seen women in which the threshold size by palpation was two or even three centimeters in diameter. The exact frequency of the above scenario is not known, but I suspect that it is more common than one might suppose. If one were to study a group of women with a complaint of a delay in diagnosis of breast cancer, I suspect that we would encounter a large number of camouflaged tumors. The camouflaged tumor should not, in my opinion, be the basis for a malpractice suit.

SUMMARY

There is an enormous variation in the threshold size of breast cancers by both mammography and palpation, as table 5–1 indicates.

Thus, under certain circumstances the presence of a fairly large tumor may be masked or camouflaged by the problems of tumor and breast density, character of tumor borders, tumor location, breast consistency, and the lack of tumor calcification. These tumors have aptly been called *camouflaged tumors*, and, as just mentioned, should not be the basis for a malpractice suit.

TABLE 5–1. DIAGNOSIS BREAST CANCER VARIATION IN THRESHOLD SIZE

EXAMINATION	CONDITIONS UNDER WHICH EXAM CONDUCTED*	
	IDEAL	ADVERSE
Mammography	2.1 to 5 mm.	2 cm. +
Palpation	3.0 to 10 mm.	2 to 3 cm.

*Takes into consideration density of the breast and tumor, breast size, etc.

REFERENCES

1. Stax P. Imaging the breast. *Surg Clin N Am* 64:1061–1072, 1984.
2. Fisher E. The impact of pathology on the biologic, diagnostic, prognostic, and therapeutic considerations in breast cancer. *Surg Clin N Am* 64(6):1073–1093, 1984.
3. Underwood JCE. A morphometric analysis of human breast carcinoma. *Br J Cancer* 26:234–237, 1972.
4. Liotta LA. Mechanism of tumor invasion. In *Important Advances in Oncology—1985*. Devita, Hellman, and Rosenberg, eds. JB Lippincott, 1985, pp. 28–41.
5. Zuckerman HC. Management of diseases of the breast. In *The Breast*. Gallager, Leis, Synderman, and Urban, eds. CV Mosby, 1978, p. 107.
6. Holland R. So-called interval cancers of the breast. *Cancer* 49:2527–2533, 1982.
7. Rosen PP. The pathology of breast carcinoma. In *Breast Diseases*. Harris, Hellman, Henderson, and Kinne, eds. JB Lippincott, 1987, pp. 147–209.
8. Harris JR and Hellman S. Conservation surgery and radiotherapy. In *Breast Diseases*. Harris, Hellman, Henderson, and Kinne, eds. JB Lippincott, 1987, p. 315.
9. Fisher ER. The pathology of invasive carcinoma. A syllabus derived from the findings of the National Adjuvant Breast Project (Protocol number 4). *Cancer* 36:1–86, 1975.
10. Wolfe, J. *Xeroradiography of the Breast*, 2nd ed. Charles Thomas, 1982). pp. 470–471.

6

THE INTERVAL TUMOR

When defending the physician charged with delay in diagnosis of breast cancer, the defense attorney should consider the possibility of an interval tumor. These carcinomas are rapidly growing and difficult to diagnose while still small. They should not be the basis for a malpractice suit since the problem in many cases is the biology of the carcinoma rather than physician error.

An interval tumor may be defined as a breast cancer that is diagnosed within 12 months following a negative screening examination (physical examination and mammogram). The carcinoma is often discovered by the patient herself or by a physician who did not perform the original screening examination. A number of investigators[1–4] have studied the interval tumors collected from various screening programs. These are all excellent articles and should be read by anyone seriously considering this diagnosis.

Holland and associates[2] presented an interesting and practical classification of their tumors surfacing within 12 months of a negative screening mammogram.

Holland's Classification of So-Called Interval Tumors

1. Missed Diagnosis   One-third of patients (approximately)
2. Camouflaged Tumor   One-third of patients (approximately)
3. True Interval Tumor One-third of patients (approximately)

1. Missed Diagnosis (modified from Holland[2])
    a. Observer error: A review of the previous mammograms revealed direct or indirect evidence of tumor at the last examination.
    b. Technical error: In several cases the tumor in question was found to lie outside the imaging field (usually extremely laterally or medially). It is also difficult to detect cancers located deep in the breast, against the chest wall, in women with small dense breasts.
2. Camouflaged Tumors[2]. (see chapter 5) These tumors were classified as camouflaged or masked because their size and calculated rate of growth (mitotic index) suggested that they were present in the breast at a size greater than six millimeters at the time of the last screening examination. A review of these 21 cases revealed that they were masked or hidden in the mammogram for several reasons:
    a. Ninety percent (19/21) of these women had very dense breasts.
    b. The carcinoma in the women who had soft breasts (2/21) contained carcinoma confined to the intraductal system. Intraductal tumors often do not produce a discrete mass.
    c. Fifty percent (9/21) of the tumors had invasive indistinct borders. These tumors were mostly infiltrative lobular carcinomas.
    d. Tumors with discrete well-defined borders tended to be diagnosed earlier than those with invasive borders.

Type of Tumor Border	Median Size at Time of Diagnosis
Discrete	2.4 cm.
Invasive, indistinct	4.6 cm.
Note: Modified from Holland[2]	

    e. Forty-six percent of the tumors with invasive borders still could not be seen in the mammogram at the time of surgery.
Holland clearly demonstrated that when the breast is dense and the tumor contains no calcifications, the tumor may be "invisible" in the mammogram and may not even be palpable

by the clinician until the neoplasm is one centimeter, two centimeters, three centimeters, or occasionally even larger.

3. The Interval Tumors[2]. There is an enormous variation in the doubling time of breast cancers (nine to 900 days). Since the average doubling time of a breast cancer is about 100 to 185 days, it is obvious that there will be many cancers with doubling times of much less than 100 days. Heuser and associates[5] concluded that ''. . . as many as 77 percent of all breast cancers may grow fast enough to grow from below threshold size detectable on mammograms to clinically detectable size in less than 12 months.'' Some will be capable of growing from one cell to a palpable cancer with metastases in less than 365 days. Some will be able to grow from a prethreshold size of 2.1 to five millimeters to a large tumor with systemic disease in less than 12 months. These rapidly growing aggressive cancers often metastasize early and are frequently the basis for a malpractice suit. Spratt[6,7] and others are of the opinion that these true interval tumors have identifiable properties that should enable us to recognize them. By this, I mean recognize them retrospectively from examination of the patient's chart, tumor tissue, and so on.

Spratt[6,7] states that interval tumors are distinctly different from ordinary cancers. He found interval tumors to be characterized by the following:

a. Rapid growth with short doubling times.
b. Anaplastic nuclear grade.
c. Frequently occurred in large dysplastic breasts that are difficult to examine clinically and by mammography.
d. Usually found in women under 50 years of age.
e. Often infiltrative invasive microscopic borders. Invasive indistinct borders make these lesions more difficult to palpate.
f. Frequently, the tumor contains no calcifications.

According to Spratt[6,7], this information has been accepted by some courts as refuting the idea that the alleged delay was responsible for the poor outcome. Certainly, in all situations where an adverse outcome is alleged to be secondary to a delay in diagnosis , the defense should be alert to the possibility of an interval tumor. If an interval tumor is suspected, defense counsel should conduct a diligent search for evidence that would suggest that he is dealing with a rapidly growing aggressive cancer. (See chapter 11 for a discussion of the determination of the aggressiveness of a breast cancer.)

SUMMARY

The adverse result frequently seen in women with true interval tumors is secondary to the biologic behavior of the breast cancer. The untoward outcome in women with the *camouflaged tumor* is secondary to the limitations of palpation and mammography in women with dense breasts. The unfortunate results in both of these situations are beyond the control of the physician, and neither one should be the basis for a malpractice suit.

REFERENCES

1. DeGroote MD, et al. Interval breast cancer: a more aggressive subset of breast neoplasias. *Surgery* 94(4):543–547, 1983.
2. Holland R, et al. So-called interval cancers of the breast. Pathologic and radiographic analysis of 64 cases. *Cancer* 49:2527–2533, 1982.
3. Heuser L, Spratt JS, et al. Relation between mammary cancer growth kinetics and the interval between screening. *Cancer* 43:857–862, 1979.
4. Spratt JS, Greenberg RA, and Heuser LS. Geometry, growth rates, and duration of cancer and carcinoma in situ of the breast before detection by screening. *Cancer Research* 46:970–974, 1986.
5. Heuser L. Spratt JS, and Polk HC. Growth rates of primary breast cancers. *Cancer* 43:1888–1894, 1979
6. Spratt JS, et al. Acute carcinoma of the breast. *S.G.O* 157:220–222, 1983.
7. Spratt JS. Discussion of a paper presented by DeGroote MD, et al. Interval breast cancer: a more aggressive subset of breast neoplasms. *Surgery* 94(4):543–547, 1983.

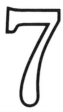

COMMON SOURCES
OF ERROR IN
CLINICAL DATA

LIMITATION OF RETROSPECTIVE STUDIES

Much of the confusion regarding the treatment of breast cancer during the past 75 years has been secondary to our reliance on the divergent findings of retrospective studies. Most retrospective studies are seriously flawed by many biases. Gelman and Zelen[1] have discussed the most common biases that plague retrospective studies.

    1. Selection bias. The selection of patients may vary from one trial to another.

    2. Eligibility bias[1,2]. Eligibility requirements for inclusion in a study may vary from trial to trial.

    3. "Stage creep" or diagnostic bias[3]. As diagnostic and staging tests improve, each stage loses patients with poor prognosis. Thus, each stage improves but the overall survival remains the same.

Stage I Stage II Stage III Stage IV	Better diagnostic tests detect patients with more extensive disease and shift them to a "worse" or higher stage. See chapter 18 for a detailed discussion of Stage Shift.

    4. Bias due to changes in definition such as tumor response, etc.

5. Bias due to differences in patient follow-up.

6. No or inadequate controls.

7. Insufficient numbers of patients in the studies.

8. Too few patients in the various subsets to permit accurate statistical analysis.

9. Other biases: lead time bias; length bias; diagnosis and over-diagnosis bias.

The only method that has been devised that will eliminate these biases is the large controlled, prospective, randomized, double blind study with at least 300 to 400 patients in each subset[1,2].

MASS SCREENING OF WOMEN WITH MAMMOGRAPHY

Prior to 1987 it was generally agreed that mass screening of asymptomatic women with mammography for breast cancer demonstrated mortality benefit only for women over the age of 50 years[2]. However, Shapiro[4] now reports that long-term follow-up of the HIP women reveals a substantial reduction in mortality for the entire group (30 percent reduction in mortality at 10 years and 25 percent reduction at 18 years). Both the 40–44 and the 45–49 age groups were found to share in this survival advantage, the 45–49 age group after five years and the 40–44 age group after eight years. Thus, it seems we now have evidence that the diagnosis and removal of small breast cancers two to three years earlier in their life cycle by mammography can reduce the long-term mortality from breast cancer.

Shapiro's report is indeed encouraging. Nevertheless, when one interprets the reports of any of the mass trials, one should be certain that the following biases have not skewed the results[1,2]:

1. Lead time bias. Periodic screening detects many cancers with occult systemic disease at an earlier stage in their life cycle. These patients live longer, thus improving the five-year survival, yet eventually die of systemic breast cancer.

2. Length bias. Slower growing tumors are more likely to be discovered by periodic screening. Faster growing tumors often surface between screens. Since slower tumors have a better survival rate, this falsely increases the overall survival.

3. Overdiagnosis bias. Periodic screening with mammography detects many small cancers with no or little lethal potential and some benign tumors that "look like" but are not cancer. This also falsely increases the survival rate.

4. Selection bias. The well-informed, intelligent woman is likely to volunteer for the screening programs. These women seem to have a higher survival rate. Why?

5. Inadequate numbers. The patients in the 40-year to 49-year age group, especially in the various subsets, limit the statistical significance of the data.

6. Classifications. The classifications of breast cancer patients according to stage, lymph node status, and tumor size are all subject to these same biases[2].

7. Some mass trials have not had control groups: for instance, the Breast Cancer Diagnosis Demonstration Project (B.C.D.D.P.).

LIMITATIONS OF MAMMOGRAPHY [5,6]

Kopans[5] has stressed: "It is important to remember that a significant number of cancers will not be detected by screening even when both physical examination as well as mammography are used." Furthermore, Kopans said that, " In the Breast Cancer Diagnosis Demonstration Project . . . almost 20 percent of the cancers were missed at screening and became clinically evident between screens (interval cancers). Based on a 100–180 day average doubling time for breast cancer, these cancers were in all probability present at the time of the screening but went undetected by the mammogram and the physical examination." (See table 7–1.) It is generally agreed that 9 to 10 percent of breast cancers (or more) cannot be visualized by mammography[6]. However, data from the B.C.D.D.P. suggest that when screening asymptomatic women, mammography may fail to detect at least 20 percent of early breast cancers[5].

TECHNICAL PROBLEMS THAT LIMIT THE EFFECTIVENESS OF MAMMOGRAPHY [5]

There are some technical problems that can limit the effectiveness of mammography in detecting a tumor:

1. The shape of the breast and its close relationship to the chest wall make it difficult to position the entire breast within the imaging fields. Some cancers may not be projected on the film.

2. When the breast is tender, it may be impossible to apply proper compression to it. All agree that the more firm the compression of the breast, the better the image in the mammogram.

3. High quality films fail to detect 10 to 15 percent of breast cancers. If the mammogram is suboptimal, the failure rate will be higher.

4. When the attenuation of the x-ray beam by the breast cancer is similar to the attenuation produced by the fibroglandular tissue of the breast, the cancer will not be visible.

5. Fat attenuates the x-ray beam much less than does a breast cancer or the normal fibroglandular structures of the breast. Thus, when a breast cancer is surrounded by fat or tissues with a high fat content, a very small cancer can be detected. (See figure 7-1.)

When the breast cancer is surrounded by fibroglandular tissue with density similar to the breast cancer, the tumor often cannot be detected by mammography. (See figure 7-2.)

Table 7-1 graphically illustrates the clinical significance and implications of the limitations of mammography.

X-Ray Beam

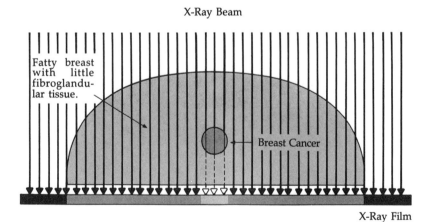

X-Ray Film

FIGURE 7-1. The breast cancer in fatty tissue. Shadow visible in film.

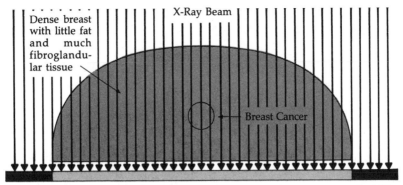

FIGURE 7–2. The breast cancer with density similar to the breast. No shadow in film.

TABLE 7–1. CLINICAL IMPLICATIONS OF THE LIMITATIONS OF MAMMOGRAPHY*

CANCER SIZE	% DIAGNOSED BY MAMMOGRAPHY	COMMENT
0.3 mm.**	0	Four years old, has developed a blood supply, begins to shed cancer cells into the blood; metastasis can and does occur [7].
2 mm.	2 to 3% +/−	Six years old, has been shedding cancer cells into the blood for about two years; metastasis can and does occur.
2 to 5 mm.	20 to 30% +/−	Six to seven years old, has been shedding cancer cells into the blood three to four years; metastasis can and does occur.
5 to 7.5 mm.	30 to 50% +/−	Shedding of cancer cells continues, metastasis can and does occur.
7.5 to 10 mm.	60 to 70% +/−	Shedding of cancer cells continues, metastasis can and does occur.
10+ mm.	85 to 90%	Eight to nine years old and 50 percent +/− has developed systemic breast cancer.

*%, years and sizes approximated.
**Size: 1 inch = 25 millimeters (mm.)
     1.2 mm. = Diameter of head of common pin.
     0.3 mm. = One-fourth the diameter of head of common pin.
     6 mm. = Diameter of the eraser on a lead pencil.

In table 7-1 we can see that by the time cancers can be detected by mammography they have been shedding cancer cells into the blood for two years or more. In some of the patients the shed cells will have produced distant metastases long before the primary cancer can be detected by mammography.

REFERENCES

1. Gelman R and Zelen M. Interpreting clinical data. In *Breast Diseases*. Harris, Hellman, Henderson, and Kinne, eds. JB Lippincott, 1987, pp 697–731.
2. Miller AB. Early detection of breast cancer. In *Breast Diseases*. Harris, Hellman, Henderson, and Kinne, eds. JB Lippincott, 1987, pp. 122–134.
3. Donegan WL. Staging and primary treatment. *Cancer of the Breast*, 3rd ed. WB Saunders, 1988, pp. 336–402.
4. Shapiro S. Determining the efficacy of breast screening. *Cancer* 63(10):1873–1880, May 15, 1989.
5. Kopans DP. The role of mammography in the diagnosis of breast cancer. In *Cancer: Principles and Practice of Oncology*, 2nd ed. Devita, Hellman, and Rosenberg, eds. (Up-date 1:(11)1–10, November 1987.)
6. Martin JE, Moskowitz M, and Milbrath J. Breast cancer missed by mammography. *Am J Radiol* 132:737–739, 1979.
7. Fisher ER. The impact of pathology on the biologic, diagnostic, prognostic and therapeutic considerations in breast cancer. *Surg Clin N Am* 64(6):1073–1093, December 1984.

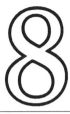

AVOID THE EARLY
DIAGNOSIS TRAP

There has been considerable controversy concerning the value of "early diagnosis" of breast cancer (see chapter 4). This is primarily a semantic debate concerning the precise definition of the word *early*. That is, just how early is an early diagnosis? Do not become involved in this controversy. Make no attempt to convince the jury that an early diagnosis is of no value. Many nationally renowned expert medical witnesses have tried and failed. Often a jury is inclined to view these efforts as an alibi for a "late" or "missed" diagnosis. With the American public's being so thoroughly indoctrinated by the American Cancer Society and media statements that an early diagnosis is synonymous with cure, it will be difficult for a jury to understand that a cure is not always possible[1]. Defense should readily agree that early diagnosis can be of value, especially early biological diagnosis. Counsel should avoid a debate concerning the value of early diagnosis and should concentrate on the following[1]:

1. Prove that the diagnosis of the plaintiff's breast cancer was timely and skillfully made. Demonstrate that the diagnosis could not have been made earlier because: either the plaintiff's breast cancer was growing more rapidly than the average breast cancer (see chapter 11); or the threshold size of the plaintiff's breast cancer was larger than the average breast cancer (see chapter 5).

2. Prove that even if the plaintiff's breast cancer had been diagnosed earlier, it is likely that the cancer had already spread systemically. Demonstrate that the plaintiff's breast cancer had a greater potential to metastasize than the average breast cancer (see chapter 11 and Appendix , section 1). Stress that tumor cells are less cohesive during cell division, and therefore rapidly growing cancers have a greater propensity to spread systemically[2]. Remind the jury that experts agree that at least 25 percent to 50 percent of breast cancers have developed systemic disease by the time the tumor has reached a diameter of 1 cm.

REFERENCES

1. Elderkin D. Personal communication, March 1988.
2. Tubiania M, et al. Kinetic parameters and the course of the disease in breast cancer. *Cancer* 47:937–943, 1981.

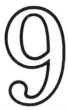

SELECTING THE MEDICAL WITNESS FOR THE DEFENSE

THE MEDICAL WITNESS FOR THE DEFENSE

Ideally, the defendant physician and the defense attorney should mutually select the expert defense witness[1,2]. This individual should possess impressive credentials for convincing the jury that he/she is truly an expert. The witness should be familiar with the growth pattern and clinical behavior of breast cancer and, in addition[1,2], should have an extensive personal experience in the diagnosis and treatment of breast cancer as well as the qualifications necessary to engage in the practice of surgical oncology. The witness should, furthermore, understand the various parameters (risk factors) that determine the risk of dying from breast cancer (see chapter 11). Finally, the witness should be familiar with the rapidly expanding literature regarding breast cancer.

THE PLAINTIFF'S EXPERT MEDICAL WITNESS

It is common knowledge that some physicians have discovered that working for a plaintiff's attorney is a lucrative source of income. If the witness is a "hired gun," the jury should be aware of this fact. During cross-examination, defense should ask:

     1. Has the witness testified in other malpractice cases? If so, how many have involved breast cancer?

2. Has the witness testified in other cases for the plaintiff's attorney? In other cases involving breast cancer for the plaintiff's attorney?

Although pathologists are experts in the diagnosis and differential diagnosis of cancer, not many have had experience or interest with the various parameters used to measure the proliferation rate and the malignant potential of breast cancer. Without experience in this area, many medical consultants tend to become confused by the conflicting opinions in the medical literature and, as a result, become ineffective in court when they try to agree with all the conflicting data[1].

We suggest that you ask your medical consultant to study this book. Obtain copies of the source material for each unfavorable risk factor found in the plaintiff's breast cancer, and encourage the pathologist and the expert witness to read these articles. The more familiar they become with this material, the more they will become convinced of the powerful predictive value of combinations of unfavorable risk factors. At the same time, they will become less concerned with the conflicting views of those inexperienced with the techniques used to measure the growth rate and malignant potential of breast cancer.

Your medical consultant must clearly understand that our goal is not only modest but realistic. We are not attempting to prove that the growth rate of the plaintiff's breast cancer was exceedingly rapid or that it possessed overwhelming lethal potential. We are merely attempting to document that the growth rate and lethal potential of her cancer were greater than the average breast cancer. If the plaintiff's breast cancer displayed no unfavorable risk factors, we must assume that the growth rate and malignant potential of her cancer were probably within the average range. If, on the other hand, one or more unfavorable risk factors were identified in the plaintiff's breast cancer, we think the pathologist and/or the expert witness should be able to state, with a reasonable degree of medical certainty, that the woman's cancer was growing more rapidly and had a greater malignant potential than the average breast cancer.

REFERENCES

1. Elderkin, D. Personal communication.
2. Jack E. Horsley, JD. Personal communication.

10

EDUCATION OF THE JURY

The foundation upon which your defense must rest is an educated jury. Robert Hanley, a prominent trial attorney, stated, "We found the jury smiles on the side that takes the mystery out of a case" (quoted by Susan Ayala, *Wall Street Journal*, July 21, 1988)[1].

Few nonprofessionals are aware of the existence of the subset of highly lethal breast cancers that grows rapidly and produces systemic disease long before they can be detected by any known diagnostic modality. For this reason it is important that the jury receive a "mini-course" in the natural history of breast cancer. A knowledgeable jury will be more receptive to a logical defense founded on these simple biologic truths. Certainly, the jury should have a clear understanding of the milestones in the life history of the typical breast cancer, including the significance of vascularization and of shedding, as well as the point in the life cycle of the cancer at which it is usually possible to detect the tumor. Other aspects of important knowledge for the jury are: the highly lethal subset of breast cancers such as the interval cancers; the concept of biologic predetermination; the limitations of mammography and palpation of the breast (the camouflaged tumor); the significance of the term *sliding threshold size*; and correlation of the proliferation rate of a breast cancer with its lethal potential.

The basic elements of the growth pattern and clinical behavior of breast cancer can be presented effectively as a series of diagrammatic drawings on large 28-by 44-inch posterboards. These are simple to prepare and make forceful presentations, especially if the drawings are quite large. This type of visual presentation can be even more effective if small posterboards are prepared for each juror, so that , as the lawyer explains the large sketch on the easel before the jury, the members of the jury can glance from time to time at their own individual small sketches and easily follow the presentation[2]. Other items such as plastic models can be of help at times.

The defense attorney should request that these exhibits (the posterboards, plastic models, etc.) go to the jury room when the jury retires for deliberation[2].

SELECTION OF THE JURY

The education of the jury should commence the moment the trial begins, that is, during the selection of the jury[3]. Defense should make every effort to select jurors who[3]: have knowledge of women who have died from breast cancer; have knowledge of people who have had a timely diagnosis and treatment of cancer and yet have died very quickly; understand that while early diagnosis and treatment *may* mean cure, this is not true in all cases; and are aware that some cancers are fatal no matter when they are discovered.

THE OPENING STATEMENT

During the opening statement, defense should give the jury a mini-course concerning the growth pattern and clinical behavior of breast cancer[3]. A series of diagrammatic sketches on posterboards makes an effective presentation.

Once again, I want to stress that I am not a legal expert and do not know the rules governing the selection of the jury, the opening statement, posing a hypothetical question, and so on. I do know, however, that the sooner the jury learns about the growth pattern and clinical behavior of breast cancer, the better off the defense will be. If the jury receives this information early in the trial, they will know what to look for as the trial proceeds.

PREPARING AN EFFECTIVE POSTERBOARD PRESENTATION

1. Use large white posterboards (at least 28 x 44 inches).
2. Draw one diagram per posterboard.
3. Keep the diagram simple.
4. The diagram should fill the entire board.
5. Use no more than six lines, and fill the entire board.
6. Use color when appropriate.
7. The diameter of the tumor in the diagrams should always be identical to the diameter of the tumor you are discussing.
8. If you are discussing the size of a breast cancer when it first develops a blood supply, place a black dot 0.3 millimeter in diameter on a large white posterboard. Do the same for the 2 millimeter, 5 millimeter, 7.5 millimeter, and 10 millimeter tumors. This will help the jury understand why some of these lesions are difficult or even impossible to identify.
9. If you are presenting a complicated idea, use a series of posterboards as we did for the interval tumor.
10. A packet of small posterboards for each juror could be quite effective.

EXAMPLES

The following diagrams will give you some ideas for a poster-board presentation of the biology of breast cancer. If the narrator desires a prompter, a typed outline of the narration can be pasted in the corner of each posterboard.

When explaining the posterboards to the jury, it is important for the narrator to avoid using complicated terms which often confuse and even alienate the jury. All technical terms should be defined using easily understood lay language[2]. For example, let's consider the word *metastasis*.

> **Metastasis.**—As this narrator begins his definition, he should turn toward the jury and say that the word *metastasis* is derived from a Greek word that means "stand beyond." This means that a cancer cell or small cluster of cancer cells has invaded and forced its way through the wall of a small blood vessel or lymph channel. When

the cancer cells enter the blood or lymph, they are carried away by the flow of blood or lymph to distant parts of the body, such as the lymph nodes, brain, liver, lung, and bone. The cluster of cancer cells finally becomes lodged in one of the small veins or lymph channels. At this point, the cancer cells invade the wall of the small vein or lymph channel and escape into the tissues of the distant organ. Here, the cluster of cancer cells grows to form a mass of cancer tissue. This mass is called a *metastasis*. The process of spreading to the distant organ is called *metastasizing*. This is what we mean when we say a patient has systemic disease.

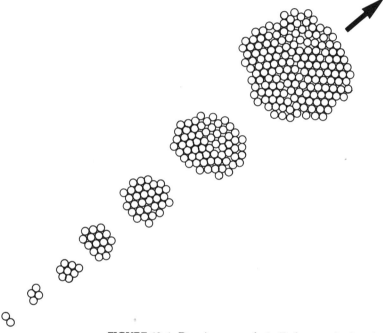

FIGURE 10–1. Drawing example 1—Early growth phase*

Narrator's Comments

1. The cancer has no blood supply during this phase of its growth.

2. The cancer cells obtain nourishment by osmosis from the surrounding tissue fluid.

3. The cancer cannot shed cells into the blood.

4. The cancer cannot metastasize.

*See text of chapter 3 for details of drawings 1–5.

Each cancer cell secretes an infiniteismal amount of a chemical called angiogenin.

The angiogenin from one or a few cells has little or no biologic effect.

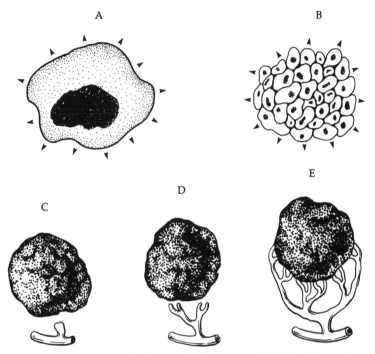

The angiogenin from thousands of tumor cells has a powerful effect. The nearby capillaries are stimulated to grow into the tumor. (C, D and E).

FIGURE 10–2. Drawing example 2—The period of vascularization.

Vital Statistics

1. When does vascularization of the tumor occur?—At about the twelfth to fourteenth net cell doubling of the tumor.

2. How many cancer cells in the tumor?—About 4,000 to 16,000 + / − .

3. How large is the tumor?—About 0.3 mm in diameter (one-fourth the size of the head of an ordinary pin).

4. How old is the tumor?—It will vary according to the doubling time of the tumor. For example, if:

Doubling time 100 days—3 1/2 years
Doubling time 60 days—2 years

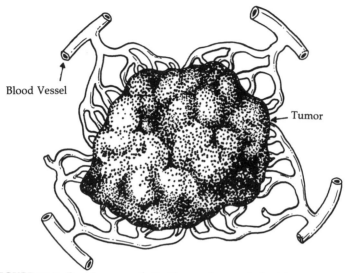

FIGURE 10–3. Drawing example 3—The newly vascularized tumor.

5. What is the significance of vascularization? Cancer cells can now escape into the blood (shedding); metastases can and do occur.

6. How do we know these things to be true? Because of studies involving implants of cancer into the vitreous of the eyes of rabbits. (The growth of the cancer can be followed with special microscopes.)

Mechanics of Cancer Growth

We measure the growth rate of a cancer by calculating the time required for the number of cancer cells within the tumor to double. For example:

1—2—4—8—16—32—64—, etc.

Unfortunately, it is not that simple. The cancer cells are dividing at a rapid pace. Many new cancer cells are being produced at the same time that many cancer cells are lost. Some individual cells or small clusters of cells die. Some cells lose their ability to reproduce. However, some cells shed into the blood.

Net Cell Doubling

A tumor contains 1,000 cancer cells, and if the net cell doubling time is 60 days, and if , in that period of 60 days: 2,000 new cancer cells are produced, and 1,000 cancer cells are lost, then the net increase of cancer cells equals 1,000. Therefore, the number of cells in the cancer has doubled, i.e., one net cell doubling has occurred. If the original tumor has 1,000 cells, and the net increase in cancer cells during a 60-day period is 1,000 cells, then after a 60-day period, the number of cells will total 2,000.

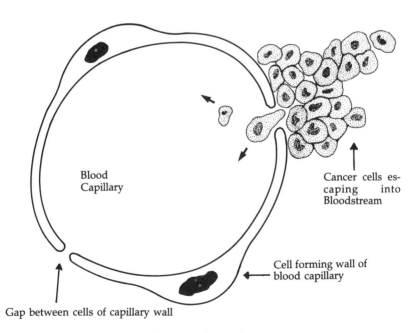

Blood Capillary

Cancer cells escaping into Bloodstream

Cell forming wall of blood capillary

Gap between cells of capillary wall

FIGURE 10–4. Drawing example 4—Shedding of cancer cells.

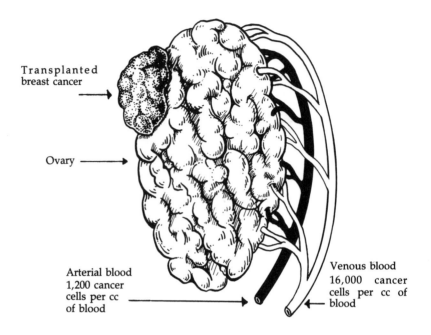

Transplanted breast cancer →

Ovary →

Arterial blood 1,200 cancer cells per cc of blood →

Venous blood 16,000 cancer cells per cc of blood ←

FIGURE 10–5. Drawing example 5—The shedding of cancer cells in an isolated rat ovary with transplanted breast cancer[4].

Note: The venous blood draining the cancerous ovary was carefully analyzed for cancer cells. From this calculation it was determined that about 3,000,000 cancer cells were shed in the venous blood every 24 hours for each gram of implanted breast cancer in the ovary (one gram equals one-fourth teaspoonful). Modified from Butler and Gullino[4].

The Fate of Shed Cancer Cells

Most shed cells die or are destroyed by the patient's immune system. Some do survive, however, since 27 percent to 50 percent of women who have a breast cancer 1 cm in diameter already have developed systemic breast cancer.

At first, the shedding of 3 million cancer cells[4] into the blood each 24 hours from a gram of tumor sounds unrealistic. However, a tumor 1 cm in diameter contains 1 billion cells, that is, 1,000 million cells. A loss of 3 million cells per day means that only one of 333 cancer cells is escaping into the blood each 24-hour period.

8–9 years old, has been shedding for about 5 to 6 years

about 7 years old, 5 to 6 mm in diameter (eraser on lead pencil is 6 mm)

about 6 years old, 2.7 mm in diameter, rarely can be seen by x-ray, has been shedding for 2 to 3 years (diameter of head of a pin is 1.2 mm)

3½ years old, 0.3 mm in diameter (one-fourth the diameter of the head of a pin), tumor has developed a blood supply and shedding and metastases can and do occur.

```
1  2  3  4  5  6  7  8  9  10  11  12  13
```

YEARS

FIGURE 10–6. Drawing example 6—Milestones in the life cycle of a breast cancer (estimated doubling time 100 days).

Notes: 1. Diagrams should always show the actual size of each cancer
2. 2.7 mm is about twice the diameter of the head of a pin
3. The vast majority of breast cancers cannot be detected until they reach a size of 5 mm or larger.
4. By the time a breast cancer reaches a detectable size it has been shedding cancer cells into the blood for at least five years.
*Source:*Modified from Gullino[7].

TABLE 10–1. RELATIONSHIP BETWEEN THE NET CELL DOUBLING, NUMBER OF CANCER CELLS, AND DIAMETER OF THE TUMOR

# NET CELL DOUBLINGS	#CELLS IN TUMOR	APPROXIMATE DIAMETER (mm)	EVENTS IN THE LIFE CYCLE OF THE TUMOR*
0	1		
9.97	1,000	0.12 mm	
13.3	10,000	0.3 mm	Vascularization of tumor
19.9	1,000,000	1.2 mm	
23.3	10,000,000	2.7 mm	Occasionally seen in x-ray

53

TABLE 10-1 (*Continued*). RELATIONSHIP BETWEEN THE NET CELL DOUBLING, NUMBER OF CANCER CELLS, AND DIAMETER OF THE TUMOR

# NET CELL DOUBLINGS	#CELLS IN TUMOR	APPROXIMATE DIAMETER (mm)	EVENTS IN THE LIFE CYCLE OF THE TUMOR*
25	100,000,000	5.8 mm	
29.9	1 billion	12.4 mm	Sometimes palpable
33.2	10 billion	26.7 mm	Common size at time of diagnosis
36	100 billion	56.6 mm	
39.9	1 trillion	124 mm	Death of host

*As interpreted by the author; see chapter 3.

Notes: cm—centimeter (1 cm–10 mm).
mm—millimeter (10 mm–1 cm).
1 inch—(2.5 cm or 25 mm).
1 billion—1,000 million.
1 trillion—1,000 billion.
Number of cells in the human body—about 11 trillion. When the number of cancer cells in a patient nears 10 percent of the total number of cells in the body (1 trillion/11 trillion), death results.

Source: Modified from: Spratt JS, et al. Geometry, growth rates, and duration of cancer and carcinoma in situ of the breast before detection by screening. *Cancer Research* 46:970, 1986. Also page 278 of Donegan and Spratt's *Cancer of the Breast*, 3rd ed., WB Saunders, 1988 [5, 6].

CANCER CELL

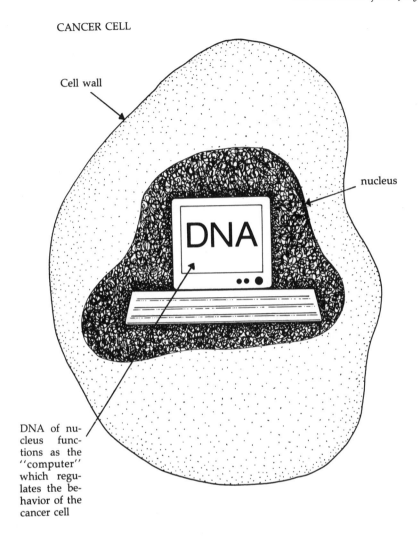

Cell wall

nucleus

DNA

DNA of nucleus functions as the "computer" which regulates the behavior of the cancer cell

FIGURE 10–7. Drawing example 7—Biologic predetermination

Narrator's Comments

The future behavior of a cancer cell is often determined by the nature of the damage to its DNA. This may occur at the moment of inception of the cancer or later as a result of an error of cell division.

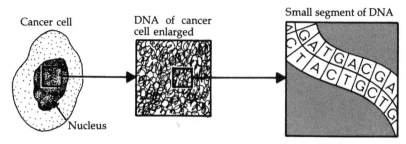

FIGURE 10–8. Drawing example 8—Biologic predetermination: The DNA of the nucleus of a cancer cell.

Narrator's Comments

1. The DNA with the nucleus consists of 46 twisted and coiled double strands of deoxyribonucleic acid.

2. When stretched out, the strands of DNA resemble a long, thin string of beads.

3. The beads are formed by four different nucleic acids which are represented by the letters T,A,C, and G.

4. The four nucleic acids (T,A,C,G) form the letters of the alphabet for the vocabulary of the genetic code of the cell's "computer." Altering one "letter" of the code can change the function of the cell.

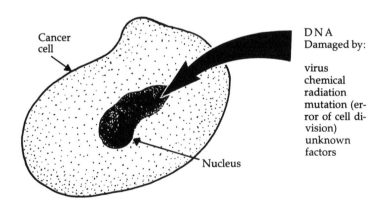

FIGURE 10–9. Drawing example 9—Biologic predetermination:The birth of a cancer cell.

5. If all of the DNA strands from all of the nuclei of one individual were stretched out and placed end to end, they would reach from the earth to the sun and back 100 times (over 20 billion miles)[8].

Narrator's Comments

1. The DNA of the nucleus may be damaged or altered by: a virus entering the nucleus; a chemical entering the nucleus; radiation; or mutation—an abnormal cell division or what some call a *mitotic aberration.* The behavior of a cancer cell may be

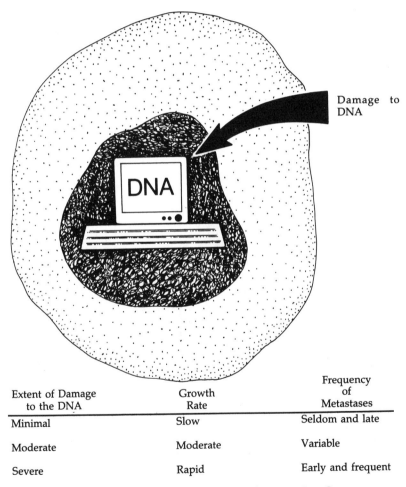

Extent of Damage to the DNA	Growth Rate	Frequency of Metastases
Minimal	Slow	Seldom and late
Moderate	Moderate	Variable
Severe	Rapid	Early and frequent

FIGURE 10–10. Drawing example 10—Biologic predetermination: Summary.

altered by a mutation at any time during its life cycle, often long before the cancer is detectable.

2. If the damaged DNA belongs to one of the genes controlling cell growth, a cancer may develop.

3. Most of the damaged cells are destroyed by the host's immune system. However, if the damaged cell escapes the immune system and is able to undergo cell division, the genetic message becomes permanent and will be passed along to all future progeny. A breast cancer has been born.

Narrator's Comments

The ultimate outcome of many breast cancers is determined by the nature of the damage to the DNA long before the tumor can be clinically detected. Twenty-seven percent to 50 percent of breast cancers have produced systemic metastases by the time the tumor reaches a diameter of one centimeter.

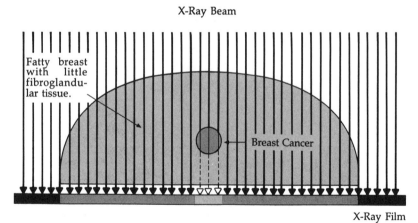

FIGURE 10–11A. Drawing example 11—Sliding threshold size. Shadow visible in film.

Note: Fat attenuates the x-ray beam much less than does a breast cancer or the normal fibroglandular structures of the breast. Thus when a cancer is situated in a breast with a high fat content a small cancer can easily be detected.

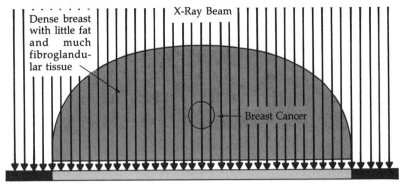

X-Ray Film

FIGURE 10–11B. Sliding threshold size. Cancer does not cast a shadow.

Note: When a breast contains little fat and is sourrounded by fibroglandular tissue with a density similar to the density of the breast cancer the tumor often cannot be visualized by mammography.

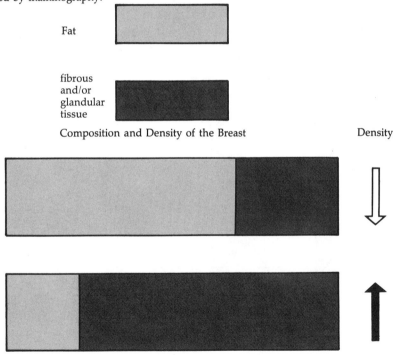

FIGURE 10–12. Drawing example 12—Density of breast also varies with composition.

Sliding Threshold Size

1 There is a wide variation in the density of both the breast and the breast cancer.

2. Therefore, it is not surprising that the density of the breast and the breast cancer is at times quite similar.

3. When the density of the breast and the breast cancer is nearly identical, it may be impossible to detect the cancer by mammography and/or palpation.

Narrator's Comments

Two factors—the marked variation in the composition and density of the tumor, and the tremendous variation in the composition and density of the breast—explain why, at times, the density of the breast and the breast tumor may be almost identical. When this occurs it will be impossible to palpate the tumor or even identify it by x-ray, providing that it contains no diagnosable tumor calcifications. This enormous variation in the tumor/breast density is why we use the term *sliding threshold size.*

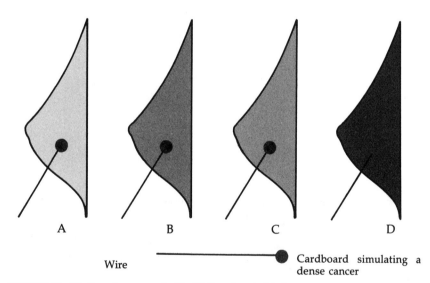

FIGURE 10—13. Drawing example 13—Sliding threshold size.

Note: In "D" the density of the tumor and the breast are nearly identical. As a result the tumor is "hidden" or camouflaged from detection by palpation and also from mammography providing the tumor contains no diagnosable calcifications.

THE INTERVAL TUMOR

Breast may be
compared to
a beaker of
water.

The surface of the water
represents the point at which
the cancer becomes clinically
detectable, i.e., the so-called
"threshold size" of the breast
cancer.

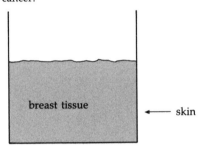

breast tissue ← skin

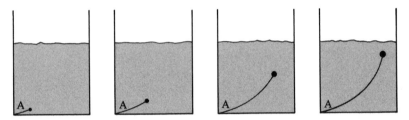

The cancer arises at point "A" and gradually increases in size

At point "B" the cancer becomes
detectable. (the threshold size)

If the cancer is not removed at
point "B" it continues to grow
from "B" towards "C".

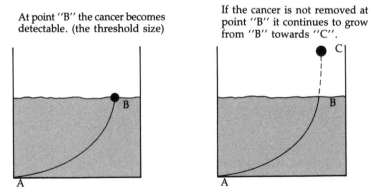

FIGURE 10–14. Drawing example 14—The interval breast cancer 1.

61

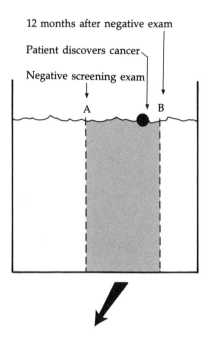

12 months after negative exam

Patient discovers cancer

Negative screening exam

A   B

Negative screening examination

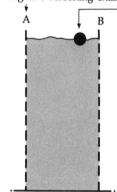

A   B

Patient discovers breast cancer

12 months following negative screening examination

The diagram on the left focuses on the 12-month period following the negative screening examination. It will help us understand the three large groups of interval breast cancers: Group A: Pure interval tumors; Group B: Interval tumors growing from a sub-threshold size of 2 to 5 mm + / – in one year; Group C: Camouflaged tumors (Figure 10–16).

FIGURE 10–15. Drawing example 15—The interval breast cancer 2.

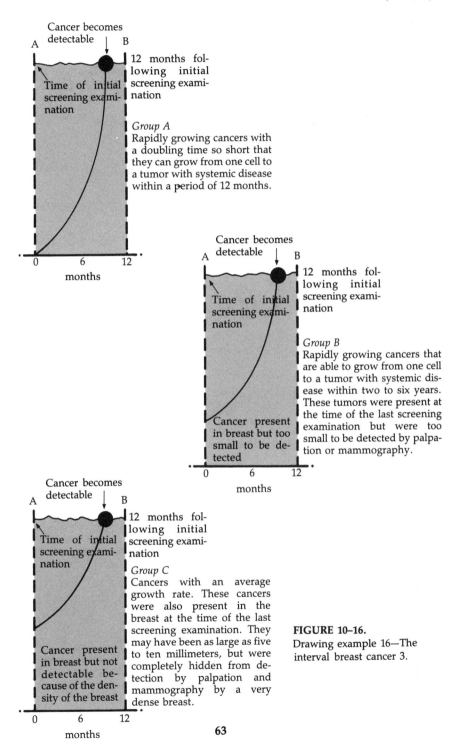

Cancer becomes detectable

A | B

12 months following initial screening examination

Time of initial screening examination

Group A
Rapidly growing cancers with a doubling time so short that they can grow from one cell to a tumor with systemic disease within a period of 12 months.

0   6   12
months

Cancer becomes detectable

A | B

12 months following initial screening examination

Time of initial screening examination

Group B
Rapidly growing cancers that are able to grow from one cell to a tumor with systemic disease within two to six years. These tumors were present at the time of the last screening examination but were too small to be detected by palpation or mammography.

Cancer present in breast but too small to be detected

0   6   12
months

Cancer becomes detectable

A | B

12 months following initial screening examination

Time of initial screening examination

Group C
Cancers with an average growth rate. These cancers were also present in the breast at the time of the last screening examination. They may have been as large as five to ten millimeters, but were completely hidden from detection by palpation and mammography by a very dense breast.

Cancer present in breast but not detectable because of the density of the breast

0   6   12
months

FIGURE 10–16.
Drawing example 16—The interval breast cancer 3.

63

TABLE 10–2. THE NET CELL DOUBLING TIME AND THE INTERVAL TUMOR

#NET CELL DOUBLINGS	# OF CELLS	
0	1	
1	2	
2	4	
3	8	
4	16	
5	32	
6	64	
7	128	
8	250 (256)*	
9	500	
10	1000	
11	2000	
12	4000	
13	8000.........Tumor develops a blood supply when it is	
14	16,000	only 0.3 mm in diameter (1/4 the size of
15	32,000	the head of a pin). Begins to shed cancer
16	64,000	cells into the blood (see chapter 3).
17	128,000	
18	250,000 (256,000)*	
19	500,000	
20	1,000,000	
21	2,000,000	
22	4,000,000......Tumor about 2 mm in diameter. In rare	
23	8,000,000	cases can be detected by x-ray if tumor
24	16,000,000	contains calcifications (head of a pin 1.2
25	32,000,000	mm) (see chapter 4).
26	64,000,00	
27	128,000,000	
28	250,000,000 (256,000,000)*...Tumor about 8.7 mm in	
29	500,000,000	diameter, the mean diameter of the first
30	1,000,000,000	mammographic shadow of the cancers
31	2,000,000,000	found in the B.C.D.D.B. by Spratt and Spratt [9].
32	4,000,000,000	
33	8,000,000,000	
34	16,000,000,000	
35	32,000,000,000	
36	64,000,000,000	
37	128,000,000,000	

TABLE 10–2 *(Continued).* THE NET CELL DOUBLING TIME AND THE INTERVAL TUMOR

#NET CELL DOUBLINGS	# OF CELLS
38	250,000,000,000 (256,000,000,000)*
39	500,000,000,000
40	1,000,000,000,000...Cancer now contains about 1 trillion cells, about 1/10 the number of cells in the human body. Death results.

*The number of cells in the tumor are ''rounded off'' or approximated for ease of computation.

The Screening Examination
Breast very dense—cancer not detectable

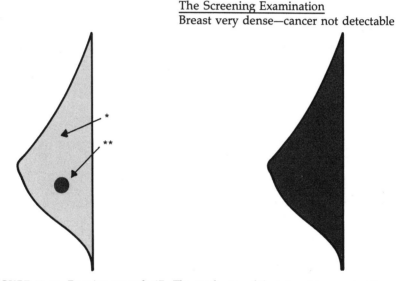

FIGURE 10–17. Drawing example 17—The mechanics of the interval tumor: An illustrative case.

* Diagram of the breast should be life-size.
** Breast cancer should be precisely 8.7 mm in diameter. Jury should be reminded that the diameter of the eraser on a pencil is 6 mm.

Narrator's Comments

How realistic is a net cell doubling time of 60 days? The average net cell doubling time of breast cancer is said to be 100 to 185 days. If the average doubling time is 142 days it is obvious that there will be many breast cancers with doubling times of much longer than 142 days and many with doubling times much shorter than 142 days. If you have discovered two or more major adverse risk factors in the plaintiff's breast cancer, a doubling time of 60 days is not at all unrealistic.

How realistic is a threshold size of 8.7 millimeters? (The threshold size is the smallest size that a tumor can be detected by the diagnostic modality under discussion.) Spratt[9] studied the breast cancers found by screening 10,000 women in the Breast Cancer Detection Demonstration Project in Louisville. He found the median threshold size of these cancers by mammography (even in retrospect) to be 8.7 millimeters. If you have found the plaintiff's breast to be more dense than the average breast, it is reasonable to assume that the threshold size of the plaintiff's breast cancer was at least 8.7 millimeters, if not larger.

As shown in the foregoing tables and figures, it is not surprising that a high percentage of breast cancers have devel-

---

TABLE 10–3. THE MECHANICS OF THE INTERVAL TUMOR (WITH A DOUBLING TIME OF 60 DAYS)

DIAMETER CANCER	# TUMOR DOUBLINGS	# OF TUMOR CELLS	# OF CELLS DYING* OR SHED	
8.7 mm	25	800,000,000		
	+1	1.6 billion	1.6 billion	
	+2	3.2 billion	3.2 billion	
1.74 cm (17.4 mm)	+3	6.4 billion	6.4 billion	360 Days
	+4	12.8 billion	12.8 billion	
	+5	25.6 billion	25.6 billion	
3.48 cm (34.8 mm)	+6	51.2 billion	51.2 billion	
⬇		⬇	⬇	
Diameter Increased 4x		# of Cells Increased 64x	The larger the tumor, the greater the number of tumor cells shed into the blood.	

*Assuming a cell loss factor of 50 percent.

oped systemic disease by the time they are large enough to be palpated. Certainly the majority of breast cancers with several or more adverse factors will have developed systemic breast cancer by the time the tumors are large enough to be detected.

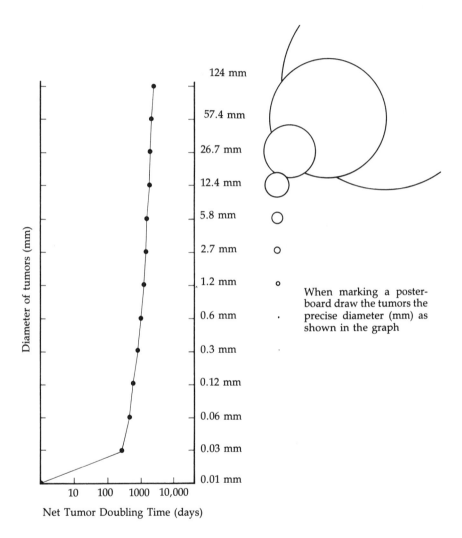

FIGURE 10–18. Drawing example 18—Net tumor volume doubling (days).
Source: Modified from Spratt et al.[5] and Spratt and Spratt[6].

REFERENCES

1. Henley. Quoted by Susan Ayala in the *Wall Street Journal,* July 21, 1988.
2. Jack E. Horsley, JD. Personal communication.
3. Elderkin, D. Personal communication, March 1988.
4. Butler PNS and Gullino PM. A quantitation of cell shedding into efferent blood of mammary adenocarcinoma. *Cancer Research* 35:512–516, 1975.
5. Spratt JS, et al. Geometry, growth rates, and duration of cancer and carcinoma in situ of the breast before detection by screening. *Cancer Research* 46:970–974, 1986.
6. Spratt JS and Spratt JA. Growth rates. In *Cancer of the Breast,* 3rd ed. Donegan and Spratt, eds. WB Saunders, 1988, p. 278.
7. Gullino PM. Natural history of breast cancer. *Cancer* 39:2697–2703, 1977.
8. de Duve, C. *A Guided Tour of the Living Cell,* vol. 2. New York: Scientific American Books Inc., p. 292.
9. Spratt JA and Spratt JS. Growth rates and the cytokinetic behavior of breast cancer. Lecture presented at the University of Heidelberg, October 1986. Personal communication.

11

ASSEMBLING THE MEDICAL FACTS FOR THE DEFENSE

A WORD OF CAUTION

I repeat, I am not an expert in legal strategy. Please do not interpret my comments as an attempt to give legal advice. The defense bar, however, should be aware of the tremendous explosion of knowledge concerning the pathophysiology of breast cancer. Not only has this resulted in dramatic changes in the treatment of breast cancer but it has explained why the unfortunate outcome of many breast cancers (the interval tumor) is often unavoidable. Therefore, when counsel is confronted with an adverse result secondary to an interval tumor, he/she must (in order to give a good defense) thoroughly understand the biology, growth pattern, and clinical behavior of breast cancer. Unfortunately, understanding is not enough. To be successful, defense must be able to communicate this information to the jury in concise and easily understood language.

My comments will be limited to the position of medical advisor. A good medical consultant should assist in the collection and analysis of all pertinent medical data.

KEEP THE OVERALL PROBLEM IN MIND

Before starting to collect our medical data, let's pause for a moment and review our overall goal and consider what we can and cannot accomplish. We must realize that because of the inherent nature of the tumor or the insensitivity of the yardsticks by which we measure tumor lethality, there will be some cases we cannot help. On the other hand, there will be many situations in which we can help, and we must remain alert to the possibility of the interval tumor, the camouflaged tumor, and the inherently lethal cancer.

An interval tumor is defined as a breast cancer that surfaces 12 months +/− following a negative screening examination which included palpation of the breast and mammography. When we examine the growth pattern of a typical interval breast cancer with a doubling time of approximately 64 days (see figure 10–18 in previous chapter[1,2]), we can easily understand the problem presented by this type of tumor. If the breast cancer is undetectable after 2.7 millimeters, there will be a serious problem.

After 5.8 millimeters, the breast cancer is rapidly increasing in size (''snowballing''). These tumors are capable of growing to an alarming size and producing systemic disease within a period of 12 to 16 months. This is especially true when the growth of the cancer is a bit more rapid than the average or when we are dealing with a breast capable of camouflaging a tumor.

From a practical standpoint, interval tumors can be divided into three groups.

One is a group of rapidly growing cancers with a net doubling time so short that it can grow from one cell to a tumor with systemic disease within 12 months (see Group A in figure 10–16, page 63).

The second group of rapidly growing cancers can grow from one cell to a tumor with systemic disease in two to six years (see Group B in figure 10–16). These tumors were present in the breast at the time of the last screening examination but were too small to be detected by palpation or mammography. That is, the tumors were present in the breast but were sub-threshold in size.

The third group of cancers has an average growth rate (Group C in figure 10–16). These cancers were also present in the breast at the time of the last screening examination. They may have been as large as 5 to 10 millimeters but were completely hidden from detection by palpation and mammography by a very dense breast. That is, they were camouflaged tumors.

Therefore, as we examine our medical data, we should be searching for two things.

1. Evidence of an increase in the growth rate or lethality of the cancer. Growth rate is important because rapidly growing tumors have a greater tendency to spread systemically before they can be detected. Some interval tumors have a rapid growth rate that can be documented by unfavorable risk factors, but other tumors with an increase are unable to be documented. Also, some interval tumors may have an average or only a slight increase in their growth rate but there may have been a camouflage problem.

2. A camouflage problem. It is well known that a dense breast can, on occasion, "hide" or conceal a breast tumor from the x-ray beam and the examining finger. Thus, the tumor will have a longer sojourn in the breast before it can be detected. This increases the likelihood of the development of systemic disease prior to detection.

Now that we have the overall objectives in mind, our first step should be to attempt to determine the malignant potential of the plaintiff's breast cancer.

DETERMINATION OF THE MALIGNANT POTENTIAL OF THE PLAINTIFF'S BREAST CANCER

Consult Your Pathologist

1. Tell your pathologist that you suspect a rapidly growing aggressive interval breast cancer.

2. Suggest that he/she read: this chapter in the manual; copies of the articles by Parl, Russo, and Bloom regarding histologic grading (see Appendix, section 2); Fisher's article regarding the predictive value of tumor nuclear grade, ER and PgR (see Appendix, section 1); and the references listed for any unfavorable risk factors discovered in the plaintiff's breast cancer (see Appendix and chapter 5).

3. Ask the pathologist to evaluate the plaintiff's breast can-

cer after he/she has read this material.

4. Have the plaintiff's tumor examined by flow cytometry. This can be done using tumor tissue from the paraffin blocks which the pathologist has in his/her possession. You will be interested in whether the S-phase fraction (percent of actively dividing cells) is high versus low and whether the DNA content is diploid or aneuploid.

5. Schedule a conference with the pathologist and discuss the results of his/her examination. Be certain that he/she has evaluated each of the following items. Many will be of no help, but you must check every item if you are to avoid overlooking a finding that would aid in establishing the malignant potential of the plaintiff's breast cancer.

Checklist for the Pathologist

> Hormone Receptors
> > Estrogen Receptor (ER)
> > Progesterone Receptor (PgR)
>
> Histologic Features
> > Nuclear Grade
> > Histologic Grade
> > Mitotic Index
>
> Microscopic Adverse Risk Factors
> > Absence of microcalcifications within the tumor
> > Infiltrative versus circumscribed pushing tumor borders
> > Vascular invasion within the tumor
> > Tumor emboli within the blood vessels in the surrounding breast
> > Lymphatic invasion or tumor emboli within the breast
> > Lymphatic invasion or tumor emboli in the beast tissue surrounding the tumor
> > Perineural lymphatic invasion
> > Focal areas of necrosis within the tumor
>
> New Tests
> > Flow cytometry
> > > S-phase fraction—high versus low
> > > DNA content—aneuploid versus diploid
> >
> > Nuclear morphometry (seldom used, consult glossary and Appendix if needed)
> > > Mean nuclear area
> > > Mitotic index (more accurate than the mitotic index determined by ordinary light microscopy)

Note: 1. Ask your pathologist to obtain the above information or to arrange for someone else to perform these data tests.
2. A DNA histogram can be obtained from archival paraffin blocks of tumor tissue. Contact: Nichols Institute
Reference Laboratories
26441 Via De Anza
San Juan Capistrano, CA 92675
1-800-LAB-TEST
1-800-522-8378
3. Some pathologists may not be familiar with the prognostic significance of some of the newer tests. If your pathologist is unable to find someone to help, contact one of the authors quoted in the sections on DNA flow cytometry or contact Nichols Institute.

Make a List of the Adverse Risk Features Found in the Plaintiff's Breast Cancer

When the list of adverse risk factors has been completed, you must establish the significance of each and demonstrate to what extent it influences the malignant potential of the plaintiff's breast cancer. To do this, the defense and the expert medical witness for the defense must consult the Appendix. The section "The Determination of the Malignant Potential of the Plaintiff's Breast Cancer; Explanation and Verification of Source Material" will supply you with the information necessary to establish the significance of the unfavorable risk factors found in the plaintiff's breast cancer. This material and the source material should be reviewed with your medical consultant.

EVALUATING THE RISK FACTORS

Hormone Receptors

The absence of an estrogen receptor (ER) or a progesterone receptor (PgR) predicts a more rapidly growing tumor with an increased risk of early recurrence. The progesterone receptor (PgR) is said to be a better predictor of prognosis than the estrogen receptor (ER).

ER − /PgR −. Twenty-seven percent of breast cancers are ER − / PgR −. If you have demonstrated the plaintiff's breast cancer to be ER – /PgR – , you have proven that her tumor was more rapidly growing and more aggressive than the breast cancers of the 40 percent of women who had ER + /PgR + breast cancers. ER – /PgR – tumors have a recurrence rate at five years that is twice that of ER + /PgR + tumors.

ER + /PgR – . Thirty percent of breast cancers are ER + /PgR – . If you have found the plaintiff's breast cancer to be ER + / PgR – , you have proven that her tumor was just as rapidly growing and aggressive as an ER – /PgR – breast cancer.

In this situation the ER is either nonfunctioning or poorly functioning. Therefore, ignore the ER status and use the PgR for your determination. (See Appendix, section 1.)

Histologic Features

- Poor nuclear grade
- Poor histologic grade (poor tubule formation)
- Frequent mitotic figures

For almost 100 years it has been known that anaplasia (immaturity of the tumor cell) and an increased number of mitotic figures (an increased rate of cell division) predict a more virulent tumor. The degree of tubule formation (histologic grade), the immaturity of the tumor nuclei (nuclear grade), and the frequency of cell division (mitotic index or grade) have been commonly used to measure the degree of anaplasia. These measurements of tumor anaplasia have never been popular since each has only a modest predictive value. Recently, however, it has been demonstrated that combinations of poor histologic grades are more powerful predictors of a poor prognosis. Combinations of poor histologic grades and low hormone receptor levels have also been shown to be powerful predictors of a high risk of recurrence of breast cancer. (See sections 1 and 2 in the Appendix for a more detailed discussion.)

If the histologic features of the plaintiff's breast cancer were classified as poor or moderately poor by the pathologist, you have proven that her tumor had a malignant potential two to two-and-a-half times greater than a tumor without these unfavorable features.

If you found combinations of unfavorable features such as:

Poor histologic grade	+	Frequent mitotic figures
	or	
Poor histologic grade	+	Poor nuclear grade

you have proven the risk of recurrence of the plaintiff's breast cancer was two to five times greater than if the breast cancer had only one unfavorable risk factor.

If you have found a tumor with a poor nuclear grade and low estrogen and progesterone levels, you have identified an aggressive breast cancer. (See sections 1 and 2 of the Appendix.)

The Adverse Microscopic Risk Factors

• Absence of microscopic calcifications within the tumor
• Infiltrative versus pushing tumor borders
• Vascular invasion within the tumor
• Tumor emboli within the blood vessels in the breast tissue surrounding the the tumor
• Lymphatic invasion or tumor emboli within the tumor
• Lymphatic invasion or tumor emboli in the breast surrounding the tumor
• Perineural lymphatic invasion
• Focal areas of necrosis within the tumor

Individually, these findings are not powerful predictors of a high rate of recurrence. However, *they are not good findings,* and they are not seen in slow-growing indolent tumors. The observation of one or more of these microscopic findings would lend credence to your contention that the plaintiff's breast cancer was indeed more aggressive than the average breast cancer. Some are better predictors than others.

Flow Cytometry

Flow cytometry is a relatively new technique but has already conclusively proven that it can provide reliable information concerning the potential lethality of a breast cancer. The flow cytometer examines and records information concerning the DNA in the nucleus of tumor cells. Tumors with an abnormal DNA content (aneuploid) versus tumors with more normal DNA (diploid) have a higher risk of relapse. Cancers whose DNA reveals a high fraction of actively dividing cells (a high S-phase fraction) also have an increased malignant potential. Flow cytometry can now be performed on tumor tissue from archival paraffin blocks, and the plaintiff's breast cancer should be examined by this technique. The results can be used in combination with hormone receptors, nuclear grade, and with the histologic grade. If the S-phase fraction is quite high, it could be used instead of the mitotic index since it is more accurate. (See the glossary for description of technique and Appendix, Section 5, for detailed discussion.)

Nuclear Morphometry

This is a seldom used but accurate method of measuring the mean nuclear diameter and area as well as calculating the mitotic index. (See the glossary for description of technique and Appendix, section 6, for complete discussion.)

A large mean nuclear area (um^2)—*u* means micron or 1/1,000 of a millimeter, um^2 means a square micron—and a high mitotic index as determined by nuclear morphometry are good predictors of prognosis.

A large mean nuclear area and/or a high mitotic index could be used in combination with other unfavorable risk factors. (See Appendix, section 6.)

Axillary Lymph Node Metastases

The presence of metastatic breast cancer in the axillary lymph nodes is a reliable predictor of systemic disease[3,4]. For example:

Axillary Lymph Nodes	*Frequency of Systemic Disease*
Negative 25–30%	These women will die
Positive 70%	of breast cancer within
	10 years

TABLE 11-1. CORRELATION BETWEEN THE NUMBER OF POSITIVE
NODES AND THE FIVE-YEAR SURVIVAL RATE OF BREAST CANCER

NUMBER OF POSITIVE NODES	FIVE-YEAR SURVIVAL
0	72%
1	63%
2	62%
3	59%
4	52%
5	47%
6–10	41%
11–15	29%

Source: Modified from Nemato et al. [5].

The presence of axillary metastases has proven to be such
an accurate predictor of systemic disease that for the past 15 to
20 years it has been the sole indication for the use of postoperative adjuvant chemotherapy for women who have axillary
lymph node metastasis (see table 11-1).

When the presence of positive lymph nodes is combined
with one or more other adverse risk factors (ER − /PgR − , poor
pathologic grade, flow cytometry, etc.), one can identify a
group of women with an extremely high risk of dying of breast
cancer.

See the appendix for a discussion of the increased predictive power of the following combinations: lymph node status,
tumor size, tumor grade and lymph node status, tumor size,
mitotic index.

A word of caution. Some may consider the presence of axillary
metastases as an indication of a delay or a "missed" diagnosis.
This, of course, is sometimes true, but more often this is simply
not the case. The regional lymph node has a biological function. It is not merely a mechanical filter for cancer cells, and
the development of nodal metastases is not a simple function
of time. Rather, the presence of metastases is a sign of a
". . . host-tumor relationship that permits the development of
metastases"[3]. In other words: the lethal potential of the tumor has overcome the resistance of the host, or the host re-

sponse was inadequate to prevent metastases from the very outset.

If you plan to employ lymph node status as an adverse risk factor, you should be prepared to present evidence of a rapidly growing tumor and/or evidence of a camouflage problem.

Tumor Size As an Adverse Risk Factor

Tumor size correlates well with survival. The larger the tumor, the greater the frequency of axillary metastases, and the higher the mortality rate (see table 11–2).

Tumor size, independent of lymph node status, is also a good predictor of outcome. The combination of lymph node status, tumor size and tumor grade or mitotic index is a potent predictor of the clinical behavior of breast cancer. See the appendix for a discussion of these combinations of risk factors.

A word of caution. Many assume that a large tumor is secondary to a "missed" diagnosis. In some instances this may be true. However, in most situations, a large tumor is secondary to one of the following: (1) a biologic predetermined rapidly growing tumor (rapid growth over a short period of time); (2) an unusually well-vascularized tumor secondary to an increased secretion of angiogenin by the tumor. These tumors can grow rapidly; and (3) a camouflage problem that has increased the threshold size of the breast cancer (see chapters 5 and 13).

TABLE 11–2. TUMOR SIZE AND FREQUENCY OF LYMPH NODE METASTASES

TUMOR SIZE	AXILLARY NODE INVOLVEMENT
1 cm.	24%
1–2 cm.	34%
2–3 cm.	43%
3–4 cm.	50%
4–5 cm.	57%
5 cm.	65%

Source: Modified from Nemato et al. [5].

One should avoid using the very large tumor (6 cm+) as an unfavorable risk factor. In some series, the survival rate for the women with very large tumors improves since some of these huge tumors tend to be slow growing and seldom metastasize.

History of Recurrence

A recurrence of the plaintiff's breast cancer would suggest that her cancer has greater malignant potential than the 40 percent of women who had slow-growing indolent cancers that seldom, if ever, metastasize (see Appendix, section 8.)

Clinical Factors

The disease-free interval. A short interval between excision of the breast cancer and recurrence suggests a rapidly growing cancer.

The Doubling Time. Occasionally, serial measurements of a metastatic lesion will permit an accurate estimation of the doubling time of the tumor.

The R_1–R_2 Interval. A short time interval between the first and second recurrence (R_1–R_2 interval) suggests a rapidly growing cancer. See chapter 15 for a complete discussion of the above.

BY MAMMOGRAPHY: DID THE PLAINTIFF HAVE A CAMOUFLAGED TUMOR?

First, consult your radiologist.

Second, both the defense and the radiologist should read chapter 5 and "Limitations of Mammography" in chapter 7, as well as the section describing the "Sliding Threshold Size" in chapter 13.

Third, review the plaintiff's mammograms with the radiologist. Tell him/her that you suspect an interval tumor and that you would like to know if there might have been a problem with camouflaging of the tumor.

A Warning

The plaintiff's attorney almost certainly will label the concept of the camouflaged tumor as an alibi for a missed diagnosis. This assertion simply is not true. The camouflaging of a tumor is a well-established medical fact and is by no means uncommon. Use your posterboard sketches to demonstrate that the problem is one of density. With a series of diagrams, prove to the jury that when the densities of the breast and a tumor (without calcifications) are nearly identical, the tumor will be "invisible" by mammography. This is true even when the tumor is large enough to be palpable. These are facts:

Fifteen to 20 percent of cancers will never by visualized by mammography.
About one-fourth of occult breast cancers contain no calcifications.
Microcalcifications are frequently not found in rapidly growing breast cancers.

Checklist for the Radiologist

Ask the radiologist to comment on the following:

Evaluate the density of the breast. Was it—
  Normal?
  Slightly increased?
  Moderately increased?
  Markedly increased?
Was there distortion of the breast secondary to—
  Diffuse or asymmetric connective tissue hyperplasia (the overgrowth of connective tissue)?
  Diffuse or asymmetric glandular hyperplasia?
  Diffuse or asymmetric cystic hyperplasia?
Was the breast size a problem? Was it a—
  Small dense breast?
  Large dense breast?
Was the technique of the mammogram a problem due to—
  Poor exposure?
  Angle of beam?
  Adequate compression?
  Motion?
Was the location of the tumor a problem? Was it—
  Deep in the breast or on the undersurface of the breast?
  Peripheral? or
  Did the location of the tumor increase the threshold size?
Was there absence of microcalcifications within the tumor?
Was there lack of distortion of the normal architectural pattern of the breast?
  Of the breast tissue itself?
  Of the vascular pattern?

Was there a problem of tumor density?
> Was the density of the tumor similar to the density of the
> breast?
> Were the tumor borders indistinct and infiltrative?
> Other factors?

In addition, discuss with the radiologist the concept of the sliding threshold size. Has he/she found structural variations noted in the plaintiff's breast that significantly increase the threshold size of her breast cancer beyond that of the so-called ideal size of the average breast cancer? Could the radiologist find any other factors that would increase threshold size of the tumor (such as tumor density, lack of calcifications within the tumor, infiltrative tumor border, etc.)?

Furthermore, ask the radiologist about Wolfe's classification of the breast parenchymal tissues. X-rays are attenuated and distorted in varying degrees, as they penetrate the structures of the breast, by the different densities of the breast tissues (fat, connective tissue, and ductal tissue). Wolfe has classified the breast parenchyma based on its radiographic image[6].

Wolfe's Parenchymal Patterns

N 1 (Normal). This breast is composed almost entirely of fat. It contains little connective or glandular tissue. The breast has a low density.

P 1 (Prominent ductal pattern). The glandular tissue is more prominent and there are sheaths of connective tissue surrounding the ducts and lobules. The ductal pattern, however, involves less than one-fourth of the breast. This breast is more dense than the N-1 breast.

P 2 (Prominent duct pattern). The ductal pattern involves more than one-fourth of the breast. More dense than the P-1 breast.

D Y (Dysplastic breast). The breast is involved with an abnormal overgrowth (dysplasia) of both the connective and glandular tissue (ducts and lobules). This breast is more dense than the P-2 breast.

Wolfe[7] agrees that when a breast cancer contains no diagnosable microcalcifications, the threshold size of the breast cancer will increase, along with the increasing density of the breast, as the parenchymal pattern changes from N1→P1→ P2→DY. Wolfe further states that when the breast is dense, small carcinomas can readily be obscured.

How Common Is the Dense Breast?

Hart and associates[8] studied the mammograms of breast tissue removed from 519 women who died of "non-hospital, non-natural or unexplained deaths." They used Wolfe's parenchymal patterns but classified them as follows:

Lucent (less dense).....................................N 1 and P 2 patterns
Dense...P 2 and DY patterns

These authors observed a shift in the parenchymal patterns from dense to lucent with age.

	% of Women with Dense Breast
Age	*(% approximated)*
20 to 30 years	75% +/−
30 to 40 years	50% +/−
60 + years	25% +/−

Modified from Hart et al.[8]

The statistics above demonstrate quite clearly that:

1. The dense breast is not at all uncommon.

2. Wolfe's parenchymal patterns are a good gauge of density.

3. When the breast cancer is not manifested primarily by tumor calcifications, the threshold size of a breast cancer increases dramatically with a progressive increase in breast density.

BY PALPATION: DID THE PLAINTIFF HAVE A CAMOUFLAGED TUMOR?

First, ask the defendant to read the chapter on "The Camouflaged Tumor" in this book.

Then, ask the defendant to review his/her clinical records regarding his/her examination of the plaintiff's breasts. Can he/she find or recall any features of the plaintiff's breasts that would contribute to the camouflaging of her breast tumor? Request that he/she consider each of the following:

Density of the breast:
Normal?
Slightly dense?
Moderately dense?
Markedly dense?

Consistency of the breast:
Normal?
Nodular? Diffuse or asymmetric (two dimensional thickening), localized or patchy?
Obese, large breast?

Next, you should consult your surgical witness. Review with him/her the findings of the radiologist and the defendant. Show him/her the mammograms. Ask your surgical witness if he/she observed any features in the plaintiff's mammograms or in the tumor that would tend to increase the threshold size of the plaintiff's breast cancer?

When we request that our consultants read certain sections of this book we are not suggesting how they should testify. Basically, we are using the book as a reference source of factors for them to consider. We want to know whether these factors were present. The witness must be able to state unequivocally that he/she was asked simply for an opinion and no opinion was suggested to him/her.

Summary

If, after careful study, your medical consultant has demonstrated that: (1) the plaintiff's breast cancer was growing a bit faster and had greater malignant potential than the average breast cancer; and (2) the plaintiff's breast possessed structural features that would tend to increase the threshold size of a breast cancer; and (3) the plaintiff's breast cancer surfaced within twelve to fourteen months after a negative screening examination, you should be able to produce convincing evidence that the defendant made a timely diagnosis of an interval breast cancer. Certainly, the jury should understand that the combination of a cancer's growing more rapidly than the average and a dense breast creates a situation where the tumor may easily reach a considerable size (two to three centimeters) and have spread systemically before a diagnosis is possible.

In many cases, the interval tumor is discovered by the patient. In this situation you *must* prove to the jury that the tumor was present at the time of the last screen but was sub-threshold in size.

REFERENCES

1. Spratt JS, et al. Geometry, growth rates, and duration of cancer and carcinoma in situ of the breast before detection by screening. *Cancer Res* 46:970–974, 1986.
2. Spratt JS and Spratt JA. Growth rates. In *Cancer of the Breast*, 3rd ed. Donegan and Spratt, eds. WB Saunders, 1988, p. 278.
3. Fisher ER. The impact of pathology on the biologic, diagnostic, prognostic, and therapeutic considerations in breast cancer. *Surg Clin N Am* 64(6):1073–1093, 1984.
4. Harris J and Henderson I. Natural history of breast cancer. *Breast Diseases*. Harris, Hellman, Henderson, and Kinne eds. JB Lippincott. 1987, pp. 233–258.
5. Nemato T, et al. Management and survival of female breast cancer. Results of a national survey by the American College of Surgeons. *Cancer* 45:2917–2924, 1980.
6. Wolfe N. Breast parenchymal patterns. In *Xeroradiography of the Breast*, 2nd ed. Charles C. Thomas, 1983.
7. Wolfe, N. Personal communication.
8. Hart L, et al. Age and race related changes in mammographic parenchymal patterns. *Cancer* 63:2537–2539, 1989.

12

THE DOUBLING TIME DEFENSE

A WORD OF CAUTION

Some have charged that the doubling time defense is inaccurate since it assumes that cancer cells divide at a constant rate over time. This, it is said, results in an overestimation of the pre-clinical phase of tumor growth. Recent studies suggest the doubling time of breast cancer slowly lengthens as the tumor increases in size (Gompertzian growth). As a result, many claim that calculations using the doubling time will give only a rough estimate of the age of the tumor, especially if the computations cover a span consisting of a large number of doublings. Although this claim may be true, some have found that calculations using doubling times obtained from serial measurements of metastases accurately predict the clinical course of the tumor. This suggests that extrapolations using realistic doubling times and limited to short periods of the clinical phase of breast cancer might be more accurate.

The plaintiff, not uncommonly, will employ the doubling time device in an attempt to prove that a breast cancer should have been detected 12 months prior to the time of surgical excision. Therefore, defense must understand the doubling time device, its limitations, and if necessary be prepared to use it as a defensive maneuver or counterattack.

In this chapter we will describe the steps involved in preparing a doubling time defense. A clear understanding of this device is essential for several reasons. First, if the plaintiff employs this device, this information will enable defense to examine critically the plaintiff's computations. Second, situations may arise in which this defense might be helpful (providing the doubling times were realistic and the extrapolations limited to a short period of time).

Before deciding to employ the doubling time defense, the medical witness for the defense should obtain a copy of Donegan and Spratt's *Cancer of the Breast*, third edition. The witness should note especially chapter 9, "Cell Kinetics of Breast and Breast Tumors" by John Meyer, pages 250–269[1] and chapter 10, "Growth Rates" by JS Spratt and JA Spratt, pages 270–302[2].

If we know the diameter of a tumor, the approximate number of cells within the tumor, and the net doubling time, it is possible to extrapolate backwards and determine the number of cancer cells in the tumor 12 months prior to the time of surgical excision of the cancer. From this information we can establish the diameter of the tumor.

AN ILLUSTRATION OF THE PROBLEM OF THE DOUBLING TIME DEFENSE

The plaintiff, a 40-year-old woman, consulted her physician for an annual physical examination. Palpation of the breasts and axilla were negative. Bilateral mammograms were said to be within normal limits. Eleven months later the plaintiff discovered a lump in her left breast. One month later the lump was removed and proved to be an infiltrating duct cell carcinoma 2.0 centimeters (20 millimeters) in diameter. A modified radical mastectomy was performed. Examination of the axillary lymph nodes revealed cancer in two nodes. A chest x-ray 18 months later revealed a metastatic pulmonary nodule 5.8 millimeters in diameter. (The eraser on an ordinary lead pencil is 6 millimeters in diameter.)

1. What was the size of the breast cancer at the time of the negative screening examination?

2. Could the breast cancer have been detected at that time?

3. When did the metastasis to the lung occur?

In order to answer these questions we must know the

following: the approximate net cell doubling time of the plaintiff's breast cancer, and the number of cancer cells in a breast tumor with a diameter of 2.0 centimeters (20 millimeters).

SUGGESTIONS FOR CREATING A HYPOTHETICAL QUESTION

To be effective, a hypothetical question should never take the medical witness for the defense by surprise. The physician should have helped the lawyer prepare the question. Each step in a series of hypothetical questions should be prepared and well documented by the lawyer and doctor working together as a team[3].

CALCULATING THE DOUBLING TIME OF THE PLAINTIFF'S BREAST CANCER

The net cell doubling time of breast cancer varies from 9 to 900 days, and it is generally agreed that the average doubling time is approximately 100 days to 185 days. If the average doubling time is 100 days to 185 days, it is obvious that there will be many breast cancers with doubling times of less than 100 days. How can we determine if the plaintiff's breast cancer had a short doubling time? Fortunately, there are a number of ways to assess the growth rate of a breast cancer.

Did the plaintiff's breast cancer surface with 12 months of a negative screening examination? If so, it might qualify as an interval tumor. Petr Skrabanek[4] stated that the doubling times of breast cancers found between screening examinations varied between 30 and 70 days. (See chapters 6 and 11.)

If the plaintiff's breast cancer was ER–/PgR– or ER+/PgR–, the growth rate was at least two times faster than an ER+/PgR+ breast cancer. (Forty percent of breast cancers are ER+; see Appendix, section 1.)

If DNA flow cytometry revealed the plaintiff's breast cancer to be aneuploid, her cancer was growing two to two-and-a-half times faster than a diploid breast cancer. (See Appendix, section 5.)

If the histologic grade of the plaintiff's breast cancer was unfavorable (moderate to poor), you will have demonstrated a growth rate more rapid than the average. (See Appendix, section 2.)

Histologic Grading

Tubule formation	Good	Moderate	Poor
Nuclear maturity	Good	Moderate	Poor
Mitotic figures	Infrequent	Moderate	Frequent

If the plaintiff should express doubt concerning the value of histologic grading, do the following:

1. Read the definition of the thymidine labeling index (TLI) in the glossary. This will remind you that the TLI is one of the most accurate measurements of the proliferation rate (growth rate) of breast cancer.

2. Agree that the TLI requires fresh tumor tissue and is not available in most clinical situations.

3. Stress that experienced investigators have demonstrated an excellent correlation between the TLI and the proliferation rate of breast cancer[5].

Thymidine Labeling Index (TLI)	Proliferation Rate of Breast Cancer
High TLI	High
Low TLI...	Low

Modified from Tubiana[5].

4. Stress also that investigators have found a profound correlation between the frequency of relapse and the proliferation rate (TLI) of breast cancer.

The TLI and Disease-Free Survival of Breast Cancer (72 mo.)
Proliferation Rate
(TLI)

Low	81% +/–
Medium..	56% +/–
High	43% +/–

Modified from Tubiana[5].

5. Stress also that these same investigators have found a

strong correlation between the TLI and the histologic grade of breast cancer. For example:

Proliferation Rate	Histologic Grade
High TLI	High Histologic Grade (poor tubule formation)[5,6]
High TLI	Poor Nuclear Grade[7]
High TLI	Frequent Mitotic Figures[5]

The above data confirm that in the absence of the thymidine labeling index the histologic grade (tubule formation), nuclear grade, and the frequency of mitotic figures are reliable indicators of the growth rate of breast cancer.

The finding of one or more adverse microscopic risk factors would be significant if accompanied by other unfavorable risk factors. (See Appendix, section 4.)

Recurrence of the breast cancer soon after surgical excision suggests a short doubling time (see chapter 15).

If several or more unfavorable risk factors were discovered in the plaintiff's breast cancer, you should be able to state with a reasonable degree of certainty that the plaintiff's breast cancer had a growth rate that was two to three times faster than the average breast cancer. The ER/PgR status and the DNA content of the tumor would be especially significant. *A net cell doubling time of 60 days would not be at all unreasonable.*

ESTABLISH THE NUMBER OF CELLS IN A TUMOR WITH A DIAMETER OF TWO CENTIMETERS

A breast cancer one centimeter in diameter contains approximately 1 billion cancer cells (1,000,000,000). When the diameter of a tumor doubles, its mass increases eightfold. Therefore, three net cell doublings are required to increase the tumor mass eight times and double the diameter of the breast cancer. For example: a tumor one centimeter in diameter contains 1 billion cells.

Net Cell Doublings	# Cancer Cells	Increase In Mass
0	1 billion	
1	2 billion	2x
2	4 billion	4x
3	8 billion	8x (diameter 2x)

TABLE 12–1. CALCULATIONS FOR NET CELL DOUBLINGS

ESTIMATED NET CELL DOUBLING TIME OF PLAINTIFF'S CANCER	365 ÷ DT	APPROXIMATE # OF NET CELL DOUBLINGS IN 365 DAYS
40 days	365 ÷ 40	9+
50 days	365 ÷ 50	7+
60 days	**365 ÷ 60**	**6+**
70 days	365 ÷ 70	5+
80 days	365 ÷ 80	4 1/2
90 days	365 ÷ 90	4

Thus a tumor with a diameter of 2 cm contains about 8 billion cancer cells.

COMPUTE THE NUMBER OF NET CELL DOUBLINGS IN 365 DAYS

To calculate the number of net cell doubling that would occur in 365 days, refer to table 12–1.

The breast cancer in our illustrative case would undergo six net cell doublings in one year.

HOW LARGE WAS THE PLAINTIFF'S BREAST CANCER 12 MONTHS PRIOR TO THE TIME OF SURGICAL EXCISION?

In order to answer this question we must extrapolate backwards and determine the number of cancer cells in the tumor 12 months prior to the time of surgical excision. From these data we can establish the approximate size of the tumor. In our illustration the diameter of the tumor at the time of removal was two centimeters (20 mm). Since we have demonstrated that a tumor with a diameter of two centimeters contains 8 billion cells, we will extrapolate backwards from 8,000,000,000 (8 billion) cancer cells (see table 12–2).

From table 12–2 we see that six net cell doublings (360 days) prior to the time of surgical excision the breast cancer in our illustration was about five millimeters in diameter. A breast cancer with a diameter of five millimeters and containing no

TABLE 12–2. EXTRAPOLATING BACKWARDS TO DETERMINE THE NUMBER OF CANCER CELLS IN A BREAST CANCER 365 DAYS PRIOR TO SURGICAL EXCISION

# NET CELL DOUBLINGS	# TUMOR CELLS	DIAMETER OF CANCER
0	8,000,000,000	2 cm (20 mm)
1	4,000,000,000	
2	2,000,000,000	
3	1,000,000,000	1 cm (10 mm)
4	500,000,000	
5	250,000,000	
6	125,000,000	0.5 cm (5 mm)
7	62,500,000	
8	31,250,000	
9	15,625,000	0.25 cm (2.5 mm)

calcification is usually not detectable, especially if situated in a dense breast.

If you plan to employ the doubling time defense, you will find chapters 9 and 10 in Donegan and Spratt's *Cancer of the Breast* most helpful[1,2]. Pay particular attention to Spratt's nomogram on page 278[2]. It will help you understand the correlation between the number of cancer cells, tumor volume, tumor diameter, and the net cell doublings of the tumor.

WHEN DID THE METASTASIS OCCUR?

A metastatic pulmonary nodule was discovered in the plaintiff's lung 18 months following surgical excision of the breast cancer. In order to answer this question we must know the following:

1. The size of the metastatic nodule—5.8 millimeters in diameter. The eraser of an ordinary lead pencil is 6 millimeters.
2. The number of cells in a nodule with a diameter of 5.8 millimeters—about 1000,000,000.
3. The estimated net cell doubling time of the plaintiff's breast cancer—about 60 days.
4. The number of net cell doubling times in 365 days—six.

TABLE 12–3. CALCULATIONS FOR DETERMINING THE AGE OF THE METASTIC NODULE

NUMBER OF NET CELL DOUBLINGS	NUMBER OF CANCER CELLS IN NODULE*	NUMBER OF NET CELL DOUBLINGS	NUMBER OF CANCER CELLS IN NODULE*
0	100,000,000	13	12,000
1	50,000,000	14	6,000
2	25,000,000	15	3,000
3	12,500,000	16	1,500
4	6,250,000	17	750
5	3,125,000	18	325
6	1,562,000	19	160
7	781,000	20	80
8	390,000	21	40
9	195,000	22	20
10	97,000	23	10
11	48,000	24	5
12	24,000		

*Number of cancer cells approximated.

Comment: Six net cell doublings occur each 360 days; therefore, the nodule is about four years of age. It was present in the lung at the time of the negative screening examination one year before the surgical excision of the breast cancer.

To calculate the age of the metastatic nodule, we must extrapolate backwards using the above information (see table 12–3).

The use of the doubling time remains controversial. If counsel elects to employ this device, he or she should be aware of its limitations.

WARNING

Metastatic pulmonary nodules appear magnified on the x-ray film because of the angle of the x-ray beam. The greater the distance of the nodule from the film, the greater the magnification (see figure 12–1). Your radiologist can determine the degree of magnification in your case by using an equation that includes the distance of the x-ray unit and the pulmonary nodule from the x-ray film. This is not a problem in mammography

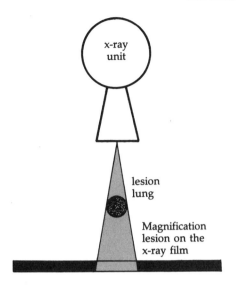

FIGURE 12–1. X-ray magnification.

because the lesions in the breast are so close to the x-ray film.

Metastases in the lung and liver often have a much shorter doubling time than the primary tumor as a result of many factors[5,8] such as increase in vascularity of the host site, increase in oxygenation of the tumor, and local immune factors. Be aware of this limitation of the use of the doubling time of metastatic lesions unless you have recorded serial measurements of the growth of the metastasis from chest x-rays, skin metastases, and so on.

CONCLUSION

We attempted to prepare a strong doubling time defense for our hypothetical case. We made a concerted effort to select a realistic doubling time and limited our extrapolations to a short period of the life cycle of the tumor. Although this may have improved the accuracy of our computations, the doubling time defense remains subject to many errors, among them:

1. The doubling time defense assumes a constant growth rate of the tumor (exponential) when actually the growth rate

is constantly decelerating (Gompertzian).

2. The arbitrary selection of a doubling time is at best a rough approximation.

3. Errors in measurement of the tumor will alter the results of your computations.

4. There may be considerable variation in the host immune surveillance over time, which may drastically affect the clinical behavior of the tumor (i.e., an indolent tumor may become aggressive)[8].

REFERENCES

1. Meyer J. Cell kinetics of breast and breast tumors. In *Cancer of the Breast*, 3rd ed. Donegan and Spratt, eds. WB Saunders, 1988, pp. 250–269.
2. Spratt JS and Spratt JA. Growth rates. In *Cancer of the Breast*, 3rd ed. Donegan and Spratt, eds. WB Saunders, 1988, pp. 270–302.
3. Jack E. Horsley, JD. Personal communication.
4. Skrabanek P. False premises and false promises of breast cancer screening. *The Lancet*, August 10, 1985, pp. 316–320.
5. Tubiana M, et al. Kinetic parameters and the course of the disease of breast cancer. *Cancer* 47:937–943, 1981.
6. Breast Flow Cytometry Study, Protocol of the North Central Cancer Treatment Group and the Mayo Clinic. October 17, 1986, p. 10.
7. Rosen PP. The pathology of breast cancer. In *Breast Diseases*. Harris, Hellman, Henderson, and Kinne, eds. JB Lippincott, 1987, pp. 147–209.
8. Gesme, D. Personal communication, May 1988.

13

THE SLIDING THRESHOLD SIZE DEFENSE

When we speak of the threshold size of a breast cancer, we like to talk of the ideal: a two millimeter cancer found in the mammogram or a one centimeter tumor discovered by palpation. Actually, there is an enormous variation in the threshold size from patient to patient. To achieve the ideal, the patient must have just the right proportion of glandular tissue, fibrous tissue, and especially fat. If there is little fat and/or an increase in glandular or fibrous tissue in the breast, the threshold size will increase dramatically. Therefore, defense should carefully review the mammograms and the clinical records to determine if there were adverse factors that would alter the threshold size. The defendant should read chapters 5 and 11 and then make a list of any adverse conditions that might have been present in the plaintiff's breast or observed in the mammogram. Were the conditions of the breast ideal? If not, were they slightly adverse or markedly adverse? The radiologist should be able to help with this determination.

The following is a brief summary of the chapter on the camouflaged tumor. Remember, the threshold is the smallest size at which a breast cancer can be detected by mammography or palpation.

THE SLIDING THRESHOLD SIZE

By Mammography
Under ideal circumstances a breast cancer occasionally may be detected by mammography when it is only two millimeters in diameter. However, most radiologists have difficulty identifying lesions smaller than five millimeters. Spratt[1] reviewed the mammograms of 232 patients in whom serial measurements of the breast cancer were available. The mean diameter of the first mammographic shadows measured 8.7 millimeters. He emphasized that most tumors in this study were detected at a larger size and only verified to be present retrospectively. Thus, in actual practice the mean threshold size for most breast cancers by mammography is about 8.7 millimeters. All agree that when several or more of the following conditions are present, the threshold size will be quite high:

1. A dense breast that contains little fat.
2. The tumor that has a density similar to the density of the breast.
3. No calcifications present within the tumor.
4. The tumor situated in certain "blind" spots (usually extremely medially or laterally).
5. The tumor that does not alter the architecture of the breast.

Under these circumstances, the tumor may not be visible until it is one centimeter, two centimeters, or even three centimeters in diameter. In about 10 to 15 percent of patients, the breast cancer will never be visible in the mammogram.

By Palpation
Under ideal circumstances, most breast cancers are palpable when they reach a diameter of one centimeter. However, this is not true when certain conditions exist in the breast: for example, when the breast is very dense and especially both dense and large; the density of the breast and the tumor are similar; and the tumor has either indistinct borders or is situated deep in the breast.

When these conditions exist, a mass of two to three centimeters may not be palpable. This reinforces a statement made by Philip Stax[2]: ''It is generally agreed that up to 20 percent of all cancers (of the breast) may not be apparent to the palpating fingers of even the most expert examiner, yet be in the early stages of a deadly disease.''

CONCLUSION

Do not let the plaintiff intimidate you. No matter how sarcastic or hostile your interrogator may be, maintain a calm demeanor. When the plaintiff insinuates that camouflaging is no more than an alibi for a missed diagnosis, stand firm. Camouflaging is a well-established medical fact. A witness not familiar with the camouflaged tumor is inexperienced in the diagnosis of breast cancer. When the plaintiff tries to impress the jury with the size of the plaintiff's breast cancer, remind the jury of the following: in the diagnosis of breast cancer it's not the actual size that is important; it's the threshold size that determines success or failure. The threshold size determines the size at

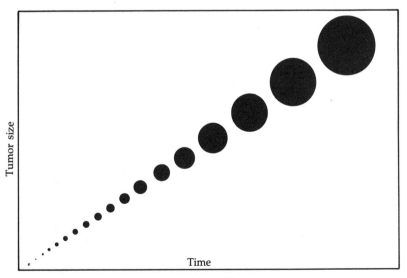

FIGURE 13–1. The sliding threshold size of breast cancer.

which it is possible to first recognize the tumor. By definition it is impossible to diagnose a subthreshold-sized tumor by any modality. Demonstrate this to the jury with the posterboard drawing shown in figure 13–1.

Instructions for Demonstrating the Sliding Threshold Size of Breast Cancer to the Jury

- Use a 28-x-44 inch posterboard
- Draw each tumor, from a black dot to 30 millimeters (3 cm), as shown. These represent a series of breast cancers. (Color should be dark gray.)
- Place the posterboard on an easel 10 or 12 feet from the jury box.
- Ask the jurors to identify the smallest dot (or cancer) that they can identify.
- Then place one large sheet of thin semi-transparent tissue paper over the posterboard.
- Again ask the jurors to identify the smallest dot (or cancer).
- Add additional sheets of tissue paper as necessary until the smallest dot that they can identify is 20 millimeters (2 cm) or larger.

This should clearly demonstrate to the jury the concept and the problems caused by the increased density of the breast secondary to excessive amounts of glandular and fibrous tissue within the breast.

REFERENCES

1. Spratt JS and Spratt JA. Growth rates and the cytokinetic behavior of breast cancer. Lecture presented at the University of Heidelberg, October 1986, personal communication.
2. Stax, P. Imaging the breast. *Surg Clin N Am* 64(6): 1061–1071, 1984.

14

DISPELLING SOME COMMON MYTHS

MYTH 1

A Large Tumor Is Evidence That the Diagnosis Was "Late" or Was a "Missed" Diagnosis

Occasionally, it is true, a large tumor may be secondary to a missed diagnosis. More commonly, however, a large tumor is secondary to one of the following:

1. A camouflage problem that has made it possible for the tumor to remain undetected for a long period of time. As mentioned previously, this frequently is the result of a very dense breast, the tumor and the breast having similar densities, the tumor having indistinct borders, the tumor being situated deep within or on the undersurface of the breast. Also, the tumor could be an infiltrating lobular carcinoma, a camouflaged infiltrating duct cell carcinoma or an intraductal carcinoma containing a small area of invasive carcinoma.

2. The tumor had a rapid growth rate.

3. The cancer was an interval tumor.

Many investigators have found the combination of lymph node status tumor size, and tumor grade of mitotic index to be a powerful predictor of prognosis. See the appendix for a complete discussion.

MYTH 2

The Presence of Axillary Lymph Node Metastases Is Usually a Sign of a "Late" Diagnosis

This statement is not true. The presence of axillary metastases is considered to be an indication of a host/tumor relationship which permitted metastases to occur.[1] (See the appendix for a discussion of the predictive power of the combination of lymph node status, tumor size, and tumor grade or mitotic index.)

MYTH 3

A Skillful Physician Would Have Detected the Plaintiff's Breast Cancer When It Was Only Two to Five Mm in Diameter

This statement is wishful thinking that ignores all the known facts. It is seldom possible to palpate a cancer smaller than ten millimeters unless it is situated on the surface of the breast of a woman with little subcutaneous fat. In this situation, it is possible to palpate a tumor three millimeters in diameter. In my own experience, this situation occurs in less than 1 percent of women (about 1/200). When the cancer is situated within the substance of the breast, it is usually impossible to palpate until it reaches a diameter of ten millimeters (1 cm). When the breast is dense or large (or both), it is often impossible to palpate a cancer until it reaches a diameter of 2 to 3.5 centimeters. In N.S.A.B.P. (National Surgical Adjuvant Breast Project) Protocol #4[1] the average size of the breast cancer when first detected was 3.4 centimeters. These women were then placed under meticulous surveillance for the early detection of a cancer in the remaining breast. This program included: (1) breast examination by a physician at six-month intervals and (2) bilateral mammogram every 12 months Patients were also encouraged to conduct monthly breast self-examinations.

In spite of this exacting follow-up routine, the average size of the cancers found in the second breast was 2.4 centimeters, only 1 centimeter smaller than the first cancer. This is stark proof that the threshold size of the breast cancers in this large group of women followed by a strict follow-up program was 2.4 centimeters.

Spratt[2] studied the breast cancers found by mammography in the Louisville B.C.D.D.P. (Breast Cancer Diagnosis Demonstration Project) which included 10,000 women. In this group of women the absolute minimum threshold size of the breast cancer was 2.2 millimeters. However, the average size of the first mammographic shadow produced by these breast cancers was 8.7 millimeters. Spratt estimated that tumors 8.7 millimeters in diameter had undergone 28 net cell doublings. He emphasized that most of these cancers were actually discovered at a larger size and verified to be visible at the 8.7 millimeter size only in retrospect.

In the day-to-day practice of medicine we must face the hard facts of reality, and sometimes this can be unpleasant. As we have demonstrated, a thoughtful scrutiny of the facts reveals that the threshold size of two millimeters by mammography and ten millimeters by palpation are merely the "ideal" and, in a practical sense, are theoretical. The true facts suggest that the average threshold size by mammography is actually about 8.7 millimeter and by palpation may be as large as 2 to 3.5 centimeters.

MYTH 4

If the Defendant Had Detected the Breast Cancer 12 Months Earlier the Plaintiff Would Have Been Cured

Not infrequently, the plaintiff will produce an "expert" witness who will testify that "if only the tumor had been removed 'x' months sooner (usually 12 months), the patient would have had an 80 to 90 percent chance of living for 10 years." In many instances this statement is unrealistic and suggests that the expert is not familiar with the current concepts of the natural history of breast cancer. We don't deny that in some cases the defendant may have been at fault, but frequently the truth is illustrated by the following scenario:

Time, zero. The plaintiff develops an invasive breast cancer, usually from one cell.

Time, three to four years +/− later. The number of tumor cells has

101

doubled about 13 to 14 times and is about one-quarter the diameter of the head of a pin (0.3 mm). (The head of a pin is about 1.2 to 2 millimeters in diameter.) It has developed a blood supply and begins shedding cancer cells into the blood.

Time, six years + / − later. The number of tumor cells has doubled about 22 times, and the tumor now is about two millimeters in diameter, which is a little larger than the head of a pin. It has been shedding cancer cells into the blood for about two years. Tumors two millimeters in diameter are rarely detected by mammography and almost never detected by palpation.

Time, seven years + / − later. The tumor is five millimeters in diameter, which is slightly smaller than the diameter of the eraser of a lead pencil. It has been shedding cancer cells into the blood for about three years.

Comment

Studies of the natural history of breast cancer have proven that the time period from the moment of inception of a breast cancer until clinical detection varies from two to 17 years. Thus, all authorities would agree that a cancer existed in the plaintiff's breast for at least two to 17 years (average six to eight years) prior to the time of diagnosis. We are suggesting that at the time of the last screening examination this tumor was two to five millimeters in diameter. Tumors of this size are usually of subthreshold size, that is, too small to be detected by mammography or by palpation of the average breast. Subthreshold tumors of this size with a growth rate that is a bit faster than the average can easily surface within 12 to 16 months as a large breast cancer with systemic disease. (For a more detailed discussion, see chapters 5, 6, and the section on the limitations of mammography in chapter 7.)

MYTH 5

The T-N-M Staging System Is Absolutely Essential for the Accurate Determination of Prognosis and the Proper Management of Breast Cancer

In actual practice most clinicians use a simple grading system that has proven to be practical and effective in the day-to-day management of breast cancer. The most frequently used staging system is described below[3].

> Stage I—The breast cancer is confined to the breast without involvement of the regional nodes or adjacent tissue.
> Stage II—The cancer has spread to the regional lymph nodes.
> Stage III—Those cases intermediate between Stage II and Stage IV
> Stage IV—Systemic disease is present.

Frequently the plaintiff's attorney will refer to the more complex T-N-M staging system (see table 14–1) and argue that the T-N-M staging system is absolutely essential to the proper diagnosis and management of breast cancer. Furthermore, he/she will assert that it is sponsored by the American College of Surgeons and the American Cancer Society and that all other systems are inadequate.

The plaintiff's attorney will always come back to the T-N-M stage at the time of the negative screening examination and compare this to the T-N-M stage at the time of the diagnosis and treatment.

When using the T-N-M staging system it is important to remember that there are two stages.

Clinical stage (cT-N-M). Based entirely upon the clinical assessment of the extent of the disease: for example, the extent of the disease at the time of the first visit.

Pathologic stage (pT-N-M). Based upon the findings at operation, the pathologic examination of the breast and regional nodes, and a clinical search for evidence of systemic disease.

AN ILLUSTRATIVE CASE

A 42-year-old woman consulted her physician regarding the possibility of a lump in her left breast. She was told that her breasts were normal and that the bilateral mammograms were negative for cancer. Eleven months later the plaintiff discovered a definite lump in her left breast.

One month later a left modified radical mastectomy was performed. Pathological examination revealed a 2.2 centimeter infiltrating duct cell carcinoma with metastasis to two lymph nodes.

TABLE 14–1. THE TNM CLASSIFICATION (1983) CURRENTLY IN USE FOR STAGING OF BREAST CANCER

I. PRIMARY TUMOR (T)

Clinical-diagnostic classification is the same as postsurgical resection—pathologic classification

TX   Minimum requirements to assess primary tumor cannot be met

TO   No evidence of primary tumor

TIS   In situ cancer (in situ lobular, pure intraductal, and Paget's disease of the nipple without palpable tumor)

Note: Paget's disease with a demonstrable tumor is classified according to size of the tumor.

Inflammatory carcinoma is reported separately. (Cancers that lack microscopic dermal lymphatic permeation are not classified as inflammatory carcinoma.)

T1÷   Tumor 2 cm or less in greatest dimension

       T1a No fixation to underlying pectoral fascia or muscle

       T1b Fixation of underlying pectoral fascia or muscle

          i. tumor $\leq$ 0.5 cm

          ii. tumor $>$ 0.5 $\leq$ 1.0 cm

          iii. tumor $>$ 1.0 $\leq$ 2.0 cm

T2+   Tumor $>$ 2 cm but not more than 5 cm in its greatest dimension

       T2a No fixation to underlying pectoral fascia or muscle

       T2b Fixation to underlying pectoral fascia or muscle

T3+   Tumor $>$ 5 cm in its greatest dimension

       T3a No fixation to underlying pectoral fascia or muscle

       T3b Fixation to underlying pectoral fascia or muscle

T4   Tumor of any size with direct extension to chest wall or skin (chest wall includes ribs, intercostal muscles, and serratus anterior muscle, but not pectoral muscle).

       T4a Fixation to chest wall

       T4b Edema (including peau d'orange), ulceration of the skin of the breast, or satellite skin nodules confined to the same breast

       T4c Both of the above

II. NODAL INVOLVEMENT (N)

Definitions for Clinical-Diagnostic Stage

NX   Regional lymph nodes cannot be assessed clinically

N0   Homolateral axillary lymph nodes not considered to contain growth

N1   Movable homolateral axillary nodes considered to contain growth

N2   Homolateral axillary nodes considered to contain growth and fixed to one another or to other structures

N3   Homolateral supraclavicular or infraclavicular nodes considered to

TABLE 14-1 *(Continued)*. **THE TNM CLASSIFICATION (1983) CURRENTLY IN USE FOR STAGING OF BREAST CANCER**

contain growth or edema of the arm (edema of the arm may be caused by lymphatic obstruction and lymph nodes may not then be palpable).

Definitions for Surgical Evaluative and Postsurgical Resection—Pathologic Stage

NX   Regional lymph nodes cannot be assessed (not removed for study or previously removed).

N0   No evidence of homolateral axillary lymph node metastasis

N1   Metastasis to movable homolateral axillary nodes not fixed to one another or to other structure

N1a   Micrometastasis $\leq$ 0.2 cm in lymph node(s)

N1b   Gross metastasis in lymph node(s)

      I Metastasis > 0.2 cm but < 2.0 cm in one to three lymph nodes

      II Metastasis > 0.2 cm but < 2.0 cm in four or more lymph nodes

      III Extension of metastasis beyond the lymph node capsule (< 2.0 cm in dimension)

      IV Metastasis in lymph node 2.0 cm or more in dimension

N2   Metastasis to homolateral axillary lymph nodes that are fixed to one another or to other structures

N3   Metastasis to homolateral supraclavicular or infraclavicular lymph node(s)

Note: Homolateral internal mammary nodes considered to contain growth are included in N3.

III. DISTANT METASTASIS (M)

MX   Minimum requirements to assess the presence of distant metastasis cannot be met.

M0   No (known) distant metastasis

M1   Distant metastasis present

STAGE GROUPING

Stage TIS In situ

Stage X   Cannot stage

Stage 1   T1ai. N0. M0

           T1aii. N0. M0

           T1aiii. N0. M0

           T1bi. N0. M0

           T1bii. N0. M0

           T1biii. N0. M0

Source: Donegan [3].

Eighteen months later 1.3 centimeters pulmonary metastasis was discovered in a routine chest x-ray.

The Plaintiff's Attorney Will Charge That . . .

The cancer should have been discovered at the time of the negative screening examination and the plaintiff should have been staged as T1-N0-M0. Proper treatment at this time would have given the plaintiff an 80 percent to 90 percent chance of living for ten years.

The pulmonary metastasis was present at the time of the negative screening examination.

The Defense Should Respond That . . .

The plaintiff's arguments contain a number of gross errors.

Error #1. The clinical stage cannot be compared to the pathological stage. They are totally different entities. We do not know the pathological stage at the time of the negative screen and we never will. However, we can be certain that a subthreshold-sized invasive cancer was present in the breast at the time of the negative screen. It could have been as large as 8.7 millimeters or even 10 millimeters or larger.

Error #2. The T-N-M staging system measures tumor burden as expressed by tumor size and lymph node status. It does not consider the inherent biologic aggressiveness of breast cancer; therefore, it is supposition to state that the plaintiff would have had an 80 percent to 90 percent chance of living for ten years.

Twenty-five percent to 30 percent of node-negative women (T1, N0, M0) will ultimately die of systemic breast cancer. Some of these high-risk women in this group might be identified by other risk factors such as low hormone receptor levels, poor histologic grade, frequent mitotic figures, DNA flow cytometry, nuclear morphometry, adverse microscopic risk factors, and so on (see appendix).

Error #3. The name *T-N-M staging system* has a nice authoritative ring to it. Actually it is seldom used since it is complex, difficult to remember, and unworkable.

Error #4. No one can determine whether, in any given case, a diagnosis was or was not timely unless he/she knows the following: the growth rate and inherent aggressiveness of the tumor; the size, density, borders, and location of the tumor;

and the size, density, borders, and location of the tumor in the breast.

REFERENCES

1. Fisher ER. The impact of pathology on the biologic, diagnostic and therapeutic considerations of breast cancer. *Surg Clin N Am* 64(6):1073–1093, 1984.
2. Spratt JS and Spratt JA. Growths rates and the cytokinetic behavior of breast cancer. Lecture presented at the University of Heidelberg, October 1986. Personal communication.
3. Donegan, William. Staging and primary treatment. In *Cancer of the Breast*, 3rd ed. Donegan and Spratt, eds. WB Saunders, 1988, pp. 336–402.

15

WHEN THE PLAINTIFF CHALLENGES THE VALIDITY OF YOUR MEDICAL DATA

INTRODUCTION

I have been told that in the past a medical expert could not be cross-examined on texts or treatises unless he/she had expressly stated in his/her examination-in-chief that he/she had relied upon those given materials in forming an opinion. It is my understanding that this has now changed and that an expert witness can now be questioned regarding the literature in all his/her areas of expertise.

Therefore, "Any expert witness should prepare himself by being certain he is familiar with all recent literature in the area in which he testifies as an expert. This should include not only articles in the reputable medical journals of established medical societies and associations but also writings in any periodical or monograph published by any reputable society comprising physicians specializing in the area in which the witness undertakes to give testimony. He may disagree with the text on which he is cross-examined. In that event, he can explain that he is familiar with the text and that he does not agree with what the writer said and that he must then be given an opportunity which might be relevant to the area in which he is giving expert testimony.''

WHEN THE PLAINTIFF CHALLENGES THE SIGNIFICANCE OF THE PREDICTIVE VALUE OF ESTROGEN AND PROGESTERONE RECEPTOR [1]

The predictive value of the estrogen receptor (ER) and the progesterone receptor (PgR) is widely accepted[1]. The witness who disagrees may be unfamiliar with the recent literature. He/she should be thoroughly questioned regarding the following:
Definition of the estrogen and progesterone receptor. Answer: a specific cytoplasmic protein that attaches to and transports estrogen and/or progesterone to the nucleus of the tumor cell where the hormone exerts its specific function. Recent evidence suggests that the estrogen receptor may normally reside within the nucleus.

The unit of measurement. Answer: the estrogen and progesterone receptors are reported as femtomoles of receptors protein per milligram of cytosol protein. Femto is a Danish word for 15, and when used as a unit of measurement it means 10^{15} or 1 quadrillionth. Mole refers to molecular weight which is the weight of a molecule of any substance representing the sum of the weights of its constituent atoms. Thus one femtomole is 1 quadrillionth of one molecular weight of the receptor protein.

Frequency of estrogen-positive breast cancer (%ER +).
Answer:

All breast cancers	50% +/−
Infiltrating duct cell carcinomas	60–70% +/−
Well-differentiated carcinomas	80–90% +/−
Lobular carcinomas	80–90% +/−

Characteristics of an estrogen-negative breast cancer. Answer: these tumors tend to have an increased proliferation rate (growth rate), an increased mitotic index (a sign of an increase in growth rate); an increased thymidine labeling index (TLI) ((which also indicates a rapidly growing tumor, and therefore anyone testifying about the growth rate of breast cancer should be familiar with it); and an increase in the recurrence rate of the cancer. Relapse of the cancer tends to occur earlier in ER- breast cancers.

WHEN THE PLAINTIFF STATES THAT THE MITOTIC INDEX HAS NO VALUE

The statement would not be true. A properly performed mitotic index performed by an experienced observer is a significant predictor of the risk of dying from breast cancer. *(See Appendix, section 2.)*

Dr. Kuhns[2] was questioned by the plaintiff's attorney concerning his experience with the mitotic index. The following is a brief summary of some of his comments.

> Average breast cancer—Dr. Kuhns finds about 3–4 mitotic figures per 10 high power fields.
> High mitotic index—Dr. Kuhns considered 5 or more mitotic figures per 10 high power fields to be a high mitotic index.
> Dr. Kuhns seldom finds more than 14–15 mitotic figures per 10 high power fields.

Some investigators (for instance, Bloom[3], Russo[4], and Parl[5]) classify their mitotic counts as follows:

Mitotic Index	# Mitotic Figures per 10 High Power Fields
Grade I (low)	0–10
Grade II (moderate)	11–20
Grade III (high)	>20

Russo[4] found no difference in the survival rate between grade II and grade III. Therefore, when considering the predictive value of the mitotic index, consider grades II and III as a single unit (high) and compare with grade I (low). How common is a high mitotic index for grades II & III?

Investigator	Frequency of a High Mitotic Index (Grades II & III)
Parl[5]*	*11/70 of patients (about 15%)
Russo[4]**	23% of his patients

*All patients had invasive duct cell carcinoma.
**All patients had infiltrating duct cell carcinoma, 135 pure duct cell, 511 mixed. Lobular and medullary excluded.

Since we have survival data for the Parl and Russo patients, it would be wise to request that your pathologist employ the technique as described by Russo for determination of the mitotic index of the plaintiff's breast cancer. (See Appendix, section 2, for a more detailed discussion of the mitotic index.)

WHEN THE PLAINTIFF CLAIMS THAT GRADING OF BREAST CANCERS ACCORDING TO THE DEGREE OF TUBULE FORMATION AND THE MATURITY OF THE TUMOR NUCLEI IS NOT A RELIABLE PREDICTOR OF MALIGNANT POTENTIAL

The plaintiff's statement is not true. Many excellent studies over the years have clearly demonstrated that the histologic grading of breast cancer is a powerful predictor of the risk of recurrence. And, as a matter of fact, of all the breast cancers, the classification of infiltrating duct cell carcinoma regarding the degree of tubule formation, nuclear maturity, and the frequency of mitoses gives the most reliable prognostic information regarding the risk of recurrence[6].

Although only several small portions of the tumor are examined, it has been proved many times that this is sufficient for an accurate evaluation of the tumor[3]. Most knowledgeable investigators now agree that if Bloom's criteria for grading are strictly followed and the grading is performed by someone with experience in this area the results will be meaningful.

In this situation the grading of infiltrating duct cell carcinoma will provide accurate information regarding the prognosis and malignant potential of the breast cancer. (See Appendix, section 2, for complete discussion of histologic grading and references for source material.)

WHEN THE PLAINTIFF CHALLENGES THE INCREASED PREDICTIVE VALUE OF COMBINATION OF ADVERSE RISK FACTORS

Parl[5] studied the predictive value of several combinations of unfavorable risk factors. For example:

Poor Tubule Formation + Frequent Mitotic Figures and
Poor Tubule Formation + Poor Nuclear Differentiation

These combinations of adverse histologic risk factors were much more powerful predictors of outcome than when used individually.

Fisher and associates[7] found combinations of ER −, PgR −, and poor nuclear grade to be more potent predictors of a poor outcome than when used alone.

Russo and associates[4] studied combinations of nuclear grade, lymph node status, ER, and tumor size. When two or three of these factors were unfavorable, the patient's risk of recurrence was extremely high.

Michael Retsky of the University of Colorado[8,9] has developed a computerized patient management system. When the patient's lymph node status, tumor size, DNA content, and treatment plan are entered into the computer, the disease-free interval for 15 years can be predicted with an accuracy of 94 percent. In the near future, Retsky plans to add the ER and PgR status to his computer program.

The above data strongly suggest that each unfavorable risk factor identifies a few high-risk women not recognized by other factors. Thus combinations of adverse risk factors become powerful predictors of an increased risk of dying from breast cancer.

WHEN THE PLAINTIFF STATES THAT FLOW CYTOMETRY IS NOT RELIABLE [10]

It is true that flow cytometry records data from benign as well as malignant cells in a breast cancer. This tends to make the S-phase fraction (the percentage of cells actively dividing) falsely low. Attempts have been made to develop computer programs that will subtract this "benign debris" from the cancer cells[10]. These programs seem to help, but the results thus far are controversial. Efforts are also in progress to develop tumor markers that will enable the cancer cells to be separated from the benign stromal cells. In the meantime the S-phase fraction of the plaintiff's breast cancer will not be of help unless it is quite high, that is, a high versus a low[11].

On the other hand, DNA flow cytometry does accurately identify and classify breast cancers according to the DNA content of the tumor nuclei. The DNA of normal cells is called diploid. Some tumor cells have a normal or near normal DNA content and will be classified as diploid by the flow cytometer.

Diploid Breast Cancers

The frequency of these cancers is about one-third of all breast cancers. The tumors are composed of benign stromal cells with normal DNA, and tumor cells with normal or near normal DNA content which will be recorded as diploid by the flow cytometer.

Aneuploid Breast Cancers

About two-thirds of breast cancers contain tumor cells that have a marked increase or decrease in the DNA content of their nuclei. Of course, they also contain benign stromal cells with normal DNA. Nevertheless, these tumors will be classified as aneuploid by the flow cytometer. Approximately 99 percent of aneuploid breast cancer cells have an increased DNA content, and 1 percent, a decreased DNA content.

Meyer[10] has stated that ". . . the probability of relapse and death within 3 years of primary treatment (of breast cancer) are increased twofold or more if the carcinoma is aneuploid rather than diploid." Thus if the plaintiff's breast cancer is aneuploid you have proven that it has more than two times the malignant potential of a diploid breast cancer.

If you are considering using DNA flow cytometry (and you should), I urge you to consult the Appendix section 5, for a complete discussion and additional references regarding the value of DNA flow cytometry.

WHEN THE PLAINTIFF CHALLENGES YOUR DATA REGARDING THE GROWTH RATE OF THE CANCER

When your data concerning the growth rate of the plaintiff's breast cancer are challenged, several steps must be taken.

Be Certain the Jury Understands That Your Goal Is Modest

First, the jury should clearly understand that you are not attempting to prove that the growth rate of the plaintiff's breast cancer was extraordinarily rapid, just more rapid than the average breast cancer and more aggressive than the average breast cancer.

Examine the Expert Witness Concerning His/Her Knowledge of the Proliferation Rate of Breast Cancer

When confronted with unfamiliar data, the natural inclination of many physicians is to challenge its validity. Thus, the data may be falsely assumed to be incorrect simply because they were unfamiliar to the physician. A truly knowledgeable witness should have no difficulty defining and/or discussing the following:

- The TLI (thymidine labeling index)
- DNA flow cytometry
  Diploid
  Tetraploid
  Aneuploid
  S-phase fraction
- Relation of the number of doubling times to the size of the tumor and the number of cancer cells in the tumor.
- Relation of tumor diameter to the number of cancer cells and tumor mass.

Prepare Your Counterattack

1. Review again the list of possible adverse risk factors (see chapter 11). Don't forget to consider lymph node status and tumor size. If possible obtain DNA flow cytometry.

2. Consult the appendix regarding each unfavorable risk

factor discovered in the plaintiff's breast cancer.

3. Review this chapter regarding the powerful predictive value of combinations of unfavorable risk factors.

4. Consult chapter 12 for a discussion of the calculation of the doubling time of a breast cancer.

Note: It is imperative that your medical witness read this material as well.

Examine the Clinical History for Indications of a Rapid Growth Rate

The disease-free interval as an indicator of the rate of growth. The disease-free interval may be defined as the interval of time between the removal of the primary tumor and the first evidence of recurrent disease. A short disease-free interval suggests a rapidly growing cancer. There are approximately 800 reported cases of untreated breast cancer in the literature[12–14]. The mean duration of life from the first symptom to death varied between 32.6 and 39.9 months. A few lived only three months while some lived for more than 30 years. A disease-free interval that is significantly shorter than three years (two years or less) would suggest a proliferation rate greater than the average breast cancer.

If there is objection to the use of the disease-free interval, you might try calculating the interval between the first symptom and the first evidence of recurrent disease. An interval of less than two years would suggest a rapidly growing tumor. If this interval were short in spite of adjuvant therapy, it would be even more significant.

The R_1-R_2 interval as an indicator of growth rat. Pearlman and Jochimsen[15] studied a group of patients with metastatic breast cancer. They defined the R_1-R_2 interval as the time interval between the first recurrence (R_1) and the second recurrence (R_2). R_1-R_2 intervals of greater than six months were classified as long and those six months or less, as short.

Interval	Median Survival
Short R^1-R_2 interval	12–16 months
Long R^1-R_2 interval	40+ months

Patients with short R_1-R_2 intervals were thought to have a greater rate of tumor progression or, in other words, these tumors were growing more rapidly. Thus, if the plaintiff's R¹-R₂ interval were six months or less, one could argue that her tumor had a growth rate more rapid than the average breast cancer.

The doubling time of metastatic lesions. If serial x-rays of metastatic lesions are available, they may be used to calculate the doubling time of the metastases. A short doubling time would suggest a rapidly growing cancer. This would be especially significant if the doubling times were short in spite of vigorous systemic treatment. Conversely, a lengthy doubling time in a woman receiving chemotherapy or hormonal therapy would have no significance.

REFERENCES

1. Harris J, Hellman S, Cannellos G, and Fisher B. Cancer of the breast. In *Cancer: Principles and Practice of Oncology*, 2nd ed. Devita, Hellman, and Rosenberg, eds. Philadelphia: JP Lippincott, 1982, p. 1150.
2. Kuhns, G., Clinical associate of pathology, University of Louisville, Louisville, KY. Testimony of the defense, District Court, Linn County, State of Iowa. *Deburkarte v. Louvar*, April 1985.
3. Bloom HJG and Richardson WW. Histologic grading and prognosis in breast cancer. *Br J Cancer* 11:359–377, 1957.
4. Russo J, et al. Predictors of recurrence and survival of patients with breast cancer. *Am J Clin Pathol* 88:123–131, 1987.
5. Parl FF, et al. A retrospective cohort study of histologic risk factors in breast cancer. *Cancer* 50:2410–2415, 1982.
6. Perez-Mesa, M. Gross and microscopic pathology. In *Cancer of the Breast*, 3rd ed. Donegan and Spratt, eds. WB Saunders, 1988, pp. 206–249.
7. Fisher B and Fisher ER, et al. Tumor nuclear grade, estrogen receptor, and progesterone receptor: their value alone or in combination as indicators of outcome following adjuvant therapy for breast cancer. *Breast Cancer Research and Treatment* 7:147–160, 1986.
8. Retsky M, et al. Prospective computerized simulation of breast cancer: comparison of computer predictions with

nine sets of biological and clinical data. *Cancer Research* 47:4982–4987, 1987.

9. Retsky, M. Quoted by Carole Bullock, *Oncology Times* 9(14), October 1988.

10. Meyer, JS. Cell kinetics of breast and breast tumors. In *Cancer of the Breast*, 3rd ed. Donegan and Spratt, eds. WB Saunders, 1988, pp. 250–269.

11. Hedley DW. Personal communication, 1988.

12. Wade P. Untreated carcinoma of the breast. *British J Radiol* 19:272, 1946.

13. Daland EM. Untreated cancer of the breast. *Surg Gyn Obst* 44:264, 1927.

14. Haagensen CD. *Disease of the Breast*. Philadelphia: WB Saunders, 1956, p. 411.

15. Pearlman NW and Jochimsen P. Recurrent breast cancer. Factors influencing survival, including treatment. *J Surg Oncol* 11:21–29, 1979.

16

WHEN THE PLAINTIFF CHARGES THAT EARLIER DETECTION WOULD HAVE MEANT LONGER LIFE

WHEN THE PLAINTIFF CHARGES THAT, IF THE BREAST CANCER HAD BEEN DETECTED 12 MONTHS EARLIER, THERE WOULD HAVE BEEN AN 80 PERCENT TO 90 PERCENT CHANCE OF LIVING FOR TEN YEARS

This statement is meaningless. It is like stating that a woman will live to be 90 years of age. Common sense tells us that this is not likely to be true unless we know the woman's age, whether she is overweight, her blood pressure, if she has diabetes, her history of alcohol and tobacco abuse, her family history of longevity, and so on.

Common sense also tells us that when we consider the ten-year survival rate of a woman with a Stage I breast cancer (axillary nodes negative), we must consider the following: the hormone receptor status of the tumor (ER + /PgR + vs ER − / PgR −); the growth rate (proliferation rate) of the breast cancer; the DNA content of the tumor nuclei (diploid versus aneu-

119

ploid); and whether adverse microscopic risk factors were found within the tumor.

Factors Influencing the Survival Rate of Stage I Breast Cancer

The hormone receptor status (ER/PgR). This status has a profound effect on the survival rate of Stage I breast cancer. An ER − stage I breast cancer has the same or even worse prognosis than an ER + Stage II breast cancer[1]. Hubay[2] reported the following:

Estrogen Receptor	Seven-Year Survival Rate
ER +	78%
ER −	63%

An ER − /PgR − Stage I breast cancer would have an even lower survival rate.

Pichon[3] reported: PgR − tumors are 3.2 times more likely to develop systemic metastases within four years than an ER + breast cancer. There is an inverse relationship between the quantitative level of PgR within the tumor and the probability of the occurrence of systemic disease. (See Appendix, section 1.) However, some dispute the clinical significance of the quanitative levels of ER and PgR, saying it does not correlate with survival.

The level of ER is less predictive of prognosis than the PgR. Combined evaluation of ER and PgR does not provide any more information than does the PgR alone.

The proliferation rate (growth rate). This factor also has a powerful effect on the survival rate of Stage I breast cancer patients. The most accurate measurement of the proliferation rate of breast cancers is the thymidine labeling index (TLI)[4].

Numerous studies have clearly demonstrated that breast cancers with a rapid proliferation rate (a high TLI) have a poor prognosis, and the higher the TLI the worse the prognosis. Unfortunately, the thymidine labeling index requires fresh tumor tissue and is, therefore, not available in most situations[4]. However, many studies have demonstrated an excellent correlation between the TLI and the following unfavorable risk factors.

- Histologic grade

Tubule formation ....moderate to poor
Nuclear maturity ....moderate to poor
Frequency of mitotic figures............moderate to frequent

- Adverse Microscopic risk factors
  See Appendix, Section 4.

Therefore, if you have found any of the above unfavorable risk factors in the plaintiff's breast cancer you have demonstrated an increase in the growth rate beyond that of the average breast cancer.

DNA flow cytometry. Fallenius and colleagues[5] have demonstrated the DNA content of Stage I breast cancer cells to be an excellent predictor of recurrence-free survival.

Stage I Breast Cancer (axillary nodes negative)	Ten-Year Recurrence-Free Survival
All patients	72%
DNA Content (Auer Classification)	
Diploid (I)	95%
Tetraploid (II)	75%
Aneuploid (III & IV)	57%

Source: Modified from Fallenius[5].

If defense can demonstrate the presence of one or more unfavorable risk factors in the plaintiff's breast cancer, you will have cast considerable doubt about the plaintiff's claim of an 80 percent to 90 percent chance of cure.

WHEN THE PLAINTIFF CHARGES THAT THE DIAGNOSIS OF HER BREAST CANCER WAS A LATE DIAGNOSIS

Almost all diagnoses of breast cancer are biologically "late." A one millimeter breast cancer (three-quarters the diameter of the head of a pin) contains 1 million cancer cells and has already undergone 20 net cell generations. Most agree that a tumor one millimeter in diameter is too small to produce symptoms or signs. Fifty percent of its life cycle is over, and yet it is too small to be detected by any currently available diagnostic modality. A ten millimeter (1 cm) breast cancer has undergone 30 net cell generations, and three-quarters of its life cycle is over. It is truly a biologically old tumor since only ten more cell generations will result in death of the host.

No one can decide whether a diagnosis was timely unless he or she understands the significance of the term *threshold size.* The threshold size of a breast cancer is the smallest size at which the tumor can be detected by the diagnostic modality under discussion. Spratt[6] found the absolute minimum threshold size of breast cancer by mammography to be 2.2 millimeter in the Louisville B.C.D.D.P.(Breast Cancer Diagnosis Demonstration Project, a mass screening of 10,000 women). The average size of the first mammographic shadow produced by the cancers found in the Louisville B.C.D.D.P. was 8.7 millimeters—this, in retrospect; most of the cancers were much larger when first detected[6].

The threshold size of breast cancer by palpation varies from three millimeters to three or more centimeters depending upon the character of the tumor and the physical composition of the woman's breast. *Therefore, no one can state that the diagnosis of a breast cancer was not timely until he/she has made an unbiased and realistic evaluation of the following:*

The density of the breast cancer
Calcifications in the tumor?
Character of the tumor border?
    Invasive versus pushing (distinct versus indistinct)
Location of the tumor within the breast
    Deep in breast
    Under surface of the breast against the chest wall?
Physical composition of the plaintiff's breast
    Very dense?
    Density of breast similar to density tumor?
    Was there a problem of patchy or diffuse overgrowth of fibrous or glandular breast tissue or mammary dysplasia?

In other words, we must establish a reasonable and honest estimate of the true threshold size of the plaintiff's breast cancer.

WHEN THE PLAINTIFF CHARGES THAT DEFENSE DOES NOT KNOW WHEN METASTASES OCCURRED

This is something that the plaintiff likes to talk about, and it is true that no one can determine the precise moment at which metastases occurs. However, we do know that metastases occurs sometime between the moment of vascularization of the tumor and the time of excision of the breast cancer. Vascularization occurs when the tumor is about three years of age. At this time the tumor has undergone 13 to 14 net cell generations (doublings), contains about 4,000 to 16,000 cancer cells, and is about 0.3 millimeters in diameter. Many investigators are of the opinion that tumors with the ability to metastasize, do so soon after the tumor becomes vascularized (see chapter 2). These investigators have established this time of metastases by calculating the doubling times of metastatic lesions from serial measurements of radiographic shadows. Then, using the number of cancer cells in the metastases (calculated from the diameter of the lesion) and the approximate doubling time of the cancer, the age of the metastasis was determined. In addition, the transplantation of breast cancer into the vitreous (eye) and the ovaries of experimental animals supports this conclusion.

Over the years it has been well documented that at least 25 percent to 50 percent of breast cancers have developed systemic breast cancer by the time the tumor is one centimeter (10 mm) in diameter.

WHEN COUNSEL CHARGES THAT THE DEFENDANT'S SCREENING INTERVALS OF THE PLAINTIFF'S BREASTS SHOULD HAVE BEEN AT SHORTER INTERVALS

The American Cancer Society, the American College of Radiology, and the American Academy of Family Physicians have recommended the following guidelines for the use of mammography[7].

1. All women with signs and symptoms of breast disease

should have mammography as well as a physical examination by a physician as often and whenever needed, regardless of age.

2. All women should have a baseline mammogram between the ages of 35 and 40 whether symptomatic or not.

3. All women between 40 and 50 should have a physical examination annually, and mammography every one, or at most, every two years.

4. All women over 50 should have both a physical examination and mammography every year.

During a trial for the alleged failure to make a timely diagnosis of an interval tumor, the plaintiff's attorney may charge that the screening intervals should have been more frequent. In order to answer this charge we must discuss the various risk factors for the development of breast cancer. The most important thing to remember about risk factors is that at least 75 percent of women who develop breast cancers do not have any evident risk factors. Thus all women must be considered at high risk for developing breast cancer[7]. For many years I faithfully recorded the risk factors of all the women who were referred with breast problems. I compiled information regarding early menarche, late menopause, age at birth of first child, number of children, nursing history, and obesity.

Each of these factors is said to be associated with a minimal and sometimes questionable increase in the risk of developing breast cancer. I cannot say that having this information ever helped me make a diagnosis of breast cancer. There are, however, some women who should be monitored more closely, and they are the following:

1. Women with a personal history of breast cancer[7]. These women have an increased risk of developing a second cancer in the remaining breast tissue. They should be followed closely through these means: monthly breast self-examinations (BSE), (with the nursing staff and/or physician reinforcing the necessity for BSE during the course of each visit); breast examination by a physician every six months; and annual mammograms, or more often if indicated.

2. Women with a family history of premenopausal breast cancer in a mother, sister or daughter have an increased risk

of developing breast cancer[7]. The risk is even higher if the mother or sister had premenopausal bilateral breast cancer. These women should be screened as above.

3. Women whose breast biopsy revealed epithelial hyperplasia with atypia[8]. These women have a significant increase in the risk of developing breast cancer, and should be screened as above.

4. Women with breast biopsies that demonstrated multiple intraductal papillomatosis[8]. These women also need a high risk screen.

5. Women whose biopsy has revealed intraductal carcinoma in situ have an increase in the risk of developing breast cancer[9–11]. These women often have multiple foci of in situ ductal carcinoma, and although not all of these lesions evolve into an invasive cancer, some do; therefore, these women should be monitored very closely with monthly BSEs, with reinforcement at each office visit; examination of the breast by a physician every four months for two years and then at six-month to twelve-month intervals as indicated; mammograms every six months for two years and then annually.

Note: A needle or core biopsy is not adequate for evaluation of this type of lesion. These lesions almost always contain microcalcifications, and therefore it is imperative that mammographic screening not be omitted.

6. Women with history of lobular carcinoma in situ also have a high risk of developing breast cancer[9,10]. These lesions are frequently multicentric and bilateral. They do not commonly contain microcalcifications and can be difficult to detect. If breast tissue remains, they should have a high-risk screen as outlined for the intraductal carcinoma in situ lesions. A needle or core biopsy is not adequate for evaluation of this type of lesion.

If the plaintiff had none of these high-risk factors, it would be difficult to make a case for a short screening interval. Some might respond that the screening interval should be more frequent for the symptomatic woman versus the asymptomatic woman. Most women have some symptoms of intermittent swelling, fullness, tenderness, sensation of lumpiness, and so on. Stax[7] is correct when he said: ''The distinction between symptomatic and asymptomatic is quite blurred." And, "In truth, every woman has breast symptoms or signs of varying severity." He goes on to say that we should consider every woman symptomatic as far as screening is concerned. Because breast cancer is often present without signs or symptoms of any kind, we should and do treat and screen all women as symptomatic whether they have symptoms or not.

Dupont and Page[12] studied the benign breast biopsies from 10,360 women who had been followed a median of 17 years. Their findings were most interesting:

1. They found virtually no difference is the absolute risk of breast cancer in the group of women with proliferative disease without atypia versus the group of women with nonproliferative breast disease. Nonproliferative disease in this study was listed as mild hyperplasia, cysts, fibroadenoma, epithelial-related calcifications, and papillary apocrine change.

2. The presence of atypia in the breast specimen increased the risk of developing breast cancer. Eight percent of the women in this group developed breast cancer within a period of 15 years.

3. A family history of breast cancer (mother, sister, or daughter) did not substantially increase the risk of breast cancer provided the breast specimen contained *no cysts and no evidence of atypia.*

4. The presence of atypia plus a family history markedly increased the risk of breast cancer. Twenty percent of these women developed breast cancer within 15 years.

The frequency of the various proliferative patterns in this large group of women was as follows:

Nonproliferative disease 69.7%
Proliferative disease 26.2%
Atypical hyperplasia..3.6%

Dupont and Page's study suggests that if a woman has a positive family history of breast cancer but the breast biopsy revealed no cysts or atypia, her risk of developing cancer of the breast will not be substantially higher than a women without a positive family history of breast cancer. This suggestion is one not generally appreciated.

REFERENCES

1. Harris J, Hellman S, Fisher B, and Canellos, GP. Cancer of the breast. In *Cancer: Principles and Practice of Oncology*, 2nd ed. Devita, Hellman, and Rosenberg, eds. JB Lippincott, 1983, p. 1150.
2. Hubay, CA. Hormone receptors, an update and application. *Surg Clin N Am* 64(6):1155–1173, 1984.
3. Pichon, M-F. Relationship of presence of progesterone receptors to prognosis in early breast cancer. *Cancer Research* 40:3357–3360, 1980.
4. Meyer JS, et al. Prediction of early course of breast cancer by thymidine labeling. *Cancer* 51:1879, 1983.
5. Fallenius AG, et al. The predictive value of nuclear DNA content of breast cancer in relation to clinical and morphologic factors. *Cancer* 62:521–530, 1988.
6. Spratt JS and Spratt JA. Growth rates and the cytokinetic behavior of breast cancer. Lecture presented at the University of Heidelberg, October 1986. Personal communication.
7. Stax, Phillip. Control of breast cancer through mass screening: from research to action. *Cancer* 63(10):1881–1887, May 1989.
8. Love S, et al. Benign breast disorders. In *Diseases of the Breast*. Harris, Hellman, Henderson, and Kinne, eds. JP Lippincott, 1987, pp. 15–53.
9. Donegan W. Staging and primary treatment. In *Cancer of the Breast*, 3rd ed. Donegan and Spratt, eds. WB Saunders, 1988, pp. 336–402.
10. Rosen PP. The pathology of breast carcinoma. In *Breast Diseases*. Harris, Hellman, Henderson, and Kinne, eds. JB Lippincott, 1987, pp. 147–209.
11. Schnitt SJ, et al. Current concepts, ductal carcinoma in situ of the breast. *N Eng J Med* 318(14):898–908, April 7, 1988.
12. Dupont WD and Page DL. Risk factors for breast cancer in women with proliferative breast disease. *N Eng J Med* 312(3):146–151, 1985.

17

HOW TO DEAL WITH THE MEDICAL WITNESS WHO IS NEVER WRONG

WHEN THE PLAINTIFF'S EXPERT WITNESS PERSISTS IN MAKING UNREALISTIC CLAIMS OF THE CURES "THAT COULD HAVE BEEN"

When the "expert" witness resolutely insists that he/she could not possibly be wrong, defense should first reread the chapter, "The Historical Perspective," as a reminder that for 75 years the rationale for the surgical treatment of breast cancer was incorrect. Second, read all the articles and lectures on breast cancer that have been authored by the "expert" witness. Has he/she performed or recommended the radical mastectomy or the modified radical mastectomy for early breast cancer? The answer should be "yes" if the witness is over the age of 40.

Questions for the Expert Witness

1. Between the years 1900 and 1975, were not the radical mastectomy and later the modified radical mastectomy the standard treatment for breast cancer?

2. Was not the rationale for these radical operations the Handley-Halsted doctrine?

3. Did not the Handley-Halsted doctrine teach the following: "Cancer of the breast spreads by direct extension through the local tissues, tissue planes, and via the lymphatics to the regional lymph nodes. When the nodes become filled the cancer spreads through the perivascular lymphatics to the bone, liver, lung, etc. Cancer of the breast seldom, if ever, spreads through the blood stream"?

4. Doctor, that was wrong, was it not?

5. Isn't it true that breast cancer spreads to the liver, bones, lungs, and brain via the blood rather than through lymphatics?

6. In fact, Doctor, cancer of the breast frequently spreads through the blood stream, does it not?

7. Doctor, if you were wrong concerning the rationale for the radical and modified radical mastectomy, how can you be certain you are not wrong now? Do you have a crystal ball? Are you psychic? (If his/her answer is "no," remind him/her that: (1) most retrospective studies are seriously biased; (2) screening trials with mammography are also marred by many biases; and much of a surgeon's clinical judgment is derived from such information as: medical school experience, postgraduate training, the medical literature he/she reads, and these are all subject to the biases of their teachers and retrospective studies. Even the surgeon's own personal surgical experience was subject to lack of controls, selection bias, insufficient numbers, and so on.

The only information not marred by these biases and limitations is data from large controlled, randomized, double blind, prospective studies; well-controlled laboratory experiments; and certain well-controlled studies of archival breast tissue. The expert witness must document the source of the data he/she is quoting and be able to prove that it is without bias. If he/she cannot, his/her testimony should be dismissed as conjecture.

The jury should be reminded that the Handley-Halsted doctrine is a classic example of how errors from retrospective studies can seriously mislead several generations of surgeons. As a result, thousands and thousands of frightened women were mutilated and defeminized by the unnecessarily radical treatment of early breast cancer. As long ago as 1922, a few brave pioneers told us this was wrong. These suggestions were refuted by the medical profession and considered to be heresy. It took surgeons 50 years to admit that they had been blinded by the countless biases that riddled the surgical literature regarding breast cancer. Now, all knowledgeable surgical oncologists and research workers realize that the Handley-Halsted doctrine was wrong.

18

PUTTING IT ALL TOGETHER

As you organize your defense you must be prepared to encounter a barrage of factual distortions and erroneous assumptions. These allegations must be promptly exposed and dispelled one by one. When the defense presents the current concepts concerning the natural history of breast cancer, you can expect the plaintiff to respond with series of clever and misleading interpretations of the facts such as:

- Defense does not believe in the value of early diagnosis because all breast cancers have systemic disease at the time of diagnosis.
- Recurrence of breast cancer suggests a "missed diagnosis."
- Breast cancers that surface within 12 months of a negative screening examination were missed at the time of the "negative screens."
- A large breast cancer (2.5 cm or larger) suggests a missed diagnosis.

It is imperative that, at the beginning of the trial, the jury learn the benefits as well as the limitations of early diagnosis. If jury members receive this information early, they will know what to look for during the course of the trial. A simple way to present the true facts concerning early diagnosis to the jury might be to compare early diagnosis with *penicillin*. Penicillin has saved more lives than any other drug in history. It is a wonderful drug, yet it has limitations and even serious side effects. Early diagnosis also can produce excellent results but it, too, has its problems.

EARLY DIAGNOSIS

Ingredients of Early Diagnosis

Important factors in diagnosing breast cancer are public education, monthly breast self-examinations, yearly breast examinations by a physician, and mammograms as indicated.

Action and Benefits

The widespread use of early diagnosis has vastly improved the ten-year survival of breast cancer (see table 18–1). Many authorities credit much of this improvement in survival to lead time bias. Nevertheless, table 18–1 graphically demonstrates that the combination of early diagnosis and radical mastectomy has produced a dramatic increase in the ten-year survival rate of breast cancer.

Limitations of Early Diagnosis

Unfortunately, there has been little or no improvement in the survival rate of breast cancer (all cases) during the past 40 to 50 years. This fact has been well documented in the medical

TABLE 18–1. THE HISTORY OF THE TREATMENT OF BREAST CANCER

	TEN-YEAR SURVIVAL RATE
250 untreated breast cancer patients, 1805–1933, Bloom	3.6%
50 radical mastectomies, 1898–1894, Halsted	32%
370 radical mastectomies, 1975, Fisher	51%

Source: Modified from Donegan [1].

literature[2–5]. Furthermore, the age-adjusted death rate of breast cancer per 100,000 female population has not decreased from 1930 to 1985 (see figure 18–1). Note from the figure the dramatic decrease in the death rate of cancer of the uterus, a marked increase in the death rate from lung cancer (women who smoke), but no decrease in the age-adjusted death from cancer of the female breast from 1930 to 1985.

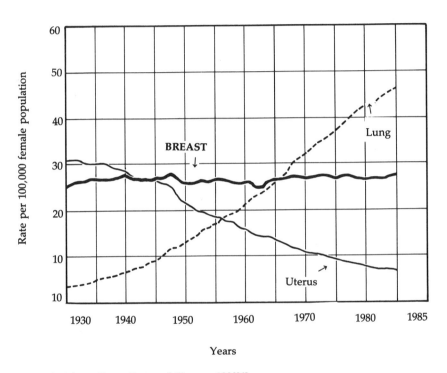

Modified from *Cancer Facts and Figures—1989*[6].
Source for data: National Center for Health Statistics and United States Bureau of the Census.

FIGURE 18–1. Age-adjusted cancer death rates for selected sites, females, United States, 1930–1982.

135

I have not been able to find age-adjusted death rates more recent than 1982. However, the five-year survival rates for female breast cancer from the American Cancer Society in 1989[7] were as follows (adjusted for normal life expectancy):

All stages..74%
Localized 90%
Regional 68%
Distant...17%

These figures sound great, and I hope they are correct. I will not be completely convinced until I see a decrease in the age-adjusted death rate from cancer of the breast.

Limitations of Treatment Programs Employing Early Diagnosis and Surgery

Procedures employed during the past 50 years include: radical mastectomy, extended radical mastectomy, modified radical mastectomy, total mastectomy with immediate or delayed axillary dissection; lumpectomy + axillary dissection + radiation to the breast. Postoperative irradiation was evaluated with each of these procedures.

In spite of the extreme variation in the extent of the breast surgery (from very radical to very conservative), the survival rate remained unchanged. How can this be true? Why does the ultraradical removal of the breast do no better than lumpectomy + axillary dissection + radiation to the breast? The answer is inescapable. In the past, 40 percent to 50 percent of women with breast cancer have had systemic disease at the time of diagnosis and treatment.

If this is true, why have there been so many reports of an increase in the survival rate of breast cancer during the past 30 to 40 years? Many factors have been responsible for creating a false impression of an increase in the survival rate of breast cancer. Among them are the following: selection bias, eligibility bias, lead time bias, length bias, overdiagnosis bias, and limitations of retrospective studies. (See chapter 7 for a complete explanation. However, the most common culprit is an illusion created by something called "stage creep" or "stage shift". When surgery is confined to increasingly favorable cases, peculiar things happen. The survival rates of both surgery and radiation improve, but the total number of patients cured remains the same! An illusion of an increased survival rate was created, while the survival actually remained the same (see table 18-2).

Should we abandon our attempts to make an early diagnosis? Absolutely not. We should continue to diagnose breast cancer as early as possible for the following reasons:

- We need to maintain the improvement in survival rates already achieved.
- We want to identify small breast cancers by mammography two to three years before they can be detected by palpation.
- Tumor resistance to chemotherapy develops over time (Goldie-Codman hypothesis), and is irrespective of tumor size or size or location of metastases. Any delay in diagnosis or treatment may risk the development of resistance to adjuvant therapy[8].
- Consider host immunity. Although little evidence has been documented, there is still considerable extrapolation of data from melanoma and renal cell carcinoma that host immunity—separate and distinct from the natural history of breast cancer cells—may change at any time for reasons

TABLE 18-2. AN EXAMPLE OF STAGE SHIFT BEFORE THE SHIFT

EXTENT DISEASE	TREATMENT	SURVIVAL	NUMBER OF CURES
I	Surgery	3/4 (75%)	3/4
II	Surgery	2/4 (50%)	2/4 } 5/8 or 63%
III	Radiation	1/4 (25%)	1/4 = 25%
	AFTER THE SHIFT		
I	Surgery	3/4 (75%)	3/4 = 75%
II	Radiation	2/4 (50%)	2/4
III	Radiation	1/4 (25%)	1/4 } 3 of 8 or 37%

Source: Modified from Donegan [1].

137

related to the cancer or entirely unrelated to it. Thus an indolent tumor could escape the host's immune control and become an aggressive cancer[8].

• We should be able to detect breast cancer at an earlier stage with continued public education, breast self-examination and mass screening programs.

THE INTERVAL TUMOR

If the history is compatible with the so-called interval tumor, defense can expect the plaintiff's attorney to respond with a charge of a missed diagnosis. The interval tumor is responsible for many unjustified malpractice suits. Why is this true? To understand, the jury must realize that there is a tremendous diversity in the biologic aggressiveness and lethal potential of breast cancer. Many have classified breast cancers as follows[9]:

• Non-metastasizing—slow growing
• Late metastasizing—intermediate growth rate and variable ability to metastasize
• Early metastasizing and rapidly growing. These early-metastasizing lesions shed cancer cells systemically almost from their inception. Examples are acute leukemia, some melanomas, and some breast cancers.

Can We Prove That These Early Metastasizing Breast Cancers Really Exist?

The answer is yes. Consider the following studies:

Koscielny and his colleagues[10] followed a large series of breast cancer patients for 10 to 25 years to determine the number that died of systemic breast cancer. They found that 40 percent of the women with breast cancers with a diameter of 2 cm ultimately died of breast cancer. This proves that 40 percent of these women had systemic breast cancer at the time of diagnosis.

Carter and associates[11] studied the survival of 24,740 women with breast cancer at the National Cancer Institute. They identified a small group of highly lethal breast cancers that were less than 5 mm in diameter. Forty-seven percent to 56 percent of these women had systemic disease at the time of diagnosis and died of breast cancer within five years.

Tinnemans and colleagues[12] studied the ten-year survival rate of female patients who had non-palpable breast cancers detected by mammography. They discovered that a significant number of these small cancers had spread systemically prior to the time of diagnosis. For example:

Size of the cancer	Number with systemic disease
5–10 mm	10% died of breast cancer
<5 mm	7.7% had positive lymph nodes

Why Does the Interval Tumor Cause So Many Problems?

Annual screening examinations (breast palpation + mammography) tend to identify the slow-growing tumors and, of course, women with this type of tumor tend to do better. The majority of the rapidly growing tumors tend to surface between screens. They were present in the breast at the time of the "negative screen" but were too small to be detected, i.e., were subthreshold in size. Many interval tumors grow fast enough to change from subthreshold size to a large tumor with metastases within a period of one year (see figure 18–2).

Figure 18–2 is an example of an interval tumor. Note the Gompertzian growth (slowly decelerating). Note also that Point A is the time of the negative screening examination, point B is 12 months following the negative screening examination, and point C is when the plaintiff discovers a lump in her breast.

The B.C.D.D.P. in Louisville screened 10,000 women annually for three years with mammography. This study identified a group of breast cancers that was growing too rapidly to permit measurement by annual mammograms[13]. These were the interval surfacing cancers. Forty-three percent of the cancers discovered in the B.C.D.D.P. mass screening trials were classified as interval tumors, that is, they surfaced within 12 months of a negative screen. Many interval cancers grow so rapidly that they can easily double their diameter twice within one year. (This requires six net cell doublings of the tumor.) A

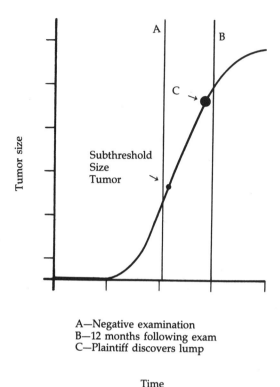

A—Negative examination
B—12 months following exam
C—Plaintiff discovers lump

Time

FIGURE 18–2. Example of the growth of an interval tumor.

subthreshold tumor with a diameter of 7 mm could easily attain a diameter of 2.8 centimeters in one year. A subthreshold tumor with a diameter of 8.7 millimeters could attain a diameter of 3.4 centimeters in one year and produce systemic disease.

The patient, of course, perceives this as a missed diagnosis, and frequently a malpractice suit results. In many of these situations the unfortunate outcome was secondary to the inherent biologic aggressiveness of the tumor. In other cases the problem was compounded by the combination of a camouflaging problem plus an aggressive tumor. This combination often proves to be lethal.

The Problem of the Camouflaged Tumor

During the course of the trial the plaintiff's attorney may charge that:

- A skillful physician would have detected this tumor because it was larger than 1 centimeter.
- The concept of the camouflaged tumor is nothing more than an alibi for a missed diagnosis.

These charges are false and should be vigorously attacked.

THE THRESHOLD SIZE BY MAMMOGRAPHY

By definition the threshold is the earliest size at which it is possible to detect a breast cancer. Each cancer has its own threshold, and these vary widely depending upon the density of the breast compared to the density of the tumor. All authorities agree that it is impossible to detect a breast cancer with a diameter less than two millimeters by mammography. The head of the common household pin is about 1.2 millimeters in diameter. During the B.C.D.D.P. screening trials in Louisville[13] 10,180 women were screened annually for three years. No breast cancer smaller than 2.1 millimeters was discovered. In the B.C.D.D.P. trial the mean diameter of the first mammographic shadow was 8.7 millimeters, and this was verified to be present only in retrospect! Thus in actual practice the average threshold size of breast by mammography was greater than 8.7 millimeters since many of these lesions were discovered only in retrospect. Of course, some cancers (at least 15 percent to 20 percent) are never visualized because the density of the tumor and the breast at times may be identical. If the tumor contains calcifications, of course, it may be detected while quite small. Thus it would not be at all unusual for a yearly screening mammogram to fail to detect an occult breast cancer with a diameter of 8.7 to 10 millimeters, providing it contained no microcalcifications. An 8.7 millimeters occult breast cancer could easily attain a diameter of 3.4 centimeters within 12 months. This would require only two doublings of the diameter of the tumor or six net cell doublings. A rapidly growing

141

interval tumor could easily accomplish this feat.

THRESHOLD SIZE BY PALPATION

It is extremely important that the jury understand the concept of the threshold size of a breast cancer. In order to convey this information effectively to the jury, defense must be thoroughly familiar with the basic facts.

Step 1

Review the following chapters: "The Camouflaged Tumor," "Assembling the Medical Facts for the Defense," and "The Sliding Threshold Size Defense."

Step 2

The jury must clearly understand that each breast cancer has a certain minimum size below which it is impossible to detect by palpation. Use the drawing in figure 10–13 shown in Chapter 10 to demonstrate to the jury the concept of the sliding threshold size. The threshold size of breast cancer is commonly said to be 1 cm. This statement, however, is very misleading since it refers to the "ideal threshold size", that is, a sharply defined tumor in a breast with normal density.

Step 3

What is the threshold size in the day-to-day practice of medicine? Donegan[14] reported that the median tumor size of 123 breast cancers with symptoms of only one to two months is 3.0 centimeters. Fisher[15] reported a large group of breast cancer patients who developed a cancer of the remaining breast during the follow-up period. The median size of the cancer in the first breast was 3.4 centimeters. During the follow-up period all women were carefully screened for the possibility of a cancer in the second breast with examination of the remaining breast every six months by a physician as well as yearly mammograms. Of course, patients were also instructed to perform monthly breast self-examinations (BSE).

In spite of this meticulous, mandated surveillance program

the median diameter of the second breast cancer was 2.4 centimeters. Many investigators have reported that many nonpalpable breast cancers found only by mammography screening programs are larger than one centimeter. Fallenius[16] reported that mean diameter of 50 nonpalpable breast cancers to be 11 millimeters. Thus, many of these cancers were much larger than 11 millimeters. Tinnemans[12] reported that 35 percent of the nonpalpable breast cancers found in his study were larger than one centimeter (10 mm). Even the most successful BSE programs fail to detect breast cancers smaller than 1.9 to 2.3 centimeters. Why, then, in actual practice, is the threshold size diameter of breast cancer by palpation so large (2 to 3 cm)? It is because of the problem of camouflaging, mentioned earlier.

Step 4

Determine the threshold size of the breast cancers found in your community. Contact the record room of your local hospital with the help of your pathologist and ask that the staff obtain the charts from the last 50 patients who had surgery for breast cancer.

Each chart should be carefully reviewed for the following: (1) the histology of each case should be identical to the plaintiff's breast cancer; and (2) each cancer should have been detected by palpation. Record the diameter of each cancer. Have the pathologist or the record room staff verify the findings.

Step 5

Consult your radiologist. Ask the radiologist to read the same chapters suggested in Step 1. Then, review the plaintiff's mammograms with the radiologist. Ask if the plaintiff's breast was more dense than the average woman's breast. Can the radiologist identify any features in the plaintiff's mammograms that might increase the threshold of a breast cancer? Ask that he or she consider the following: size of breast, density of tumor, dysplasia, density of breast, location of tumor, tumor border (was it indefinite?), and consistency of breast.

Be certain that he or she has read the section of Wolfe's classification of breast parenchymal patterns in chapter 11.

143

Could the plaintiff's breast be classified as P2 or DY?

Step 6

Consult your pathologist. Ask if he or she could find any features in the plaintiff's breast that would tend to increase the threshold size of the plaintiff's breast cancer. By *mammography,* the pathologist should be able to detect an absence of microcalcifications. *By palpation,* the following features might be detected:

- vague infiltrative tumor borders
- an infiltrating lobular carcinoma (these tumors are often camouflaged)
- an infiltrative duct cell carcinoma with a large component of intraductal carcinoma which can be difficult to palpate
- location in the breast
  -deep in the breast
  -lying against the chest wall
- density or consistency of the breast
  -dense breast
  -dysplastic breast

In addition, ask your pathologist to read chapter 5, "The Camouflaged Tumor."

Step 7

Was the plaintiff's breast cancer more aggressive than the average cancer? The T-N-M staging system gives us an estimate of the extent of the disease (the tumor burden). Unfortunately, tumor burden as measured by tumor size and lymph node status does not adequately consider the inherent biologic aggressiveness of breast cancer. As a result, it fails to identify the 30 percent to 43 percent of node-negative women who will ultimately die of breast cancer. There is a growing body of evidence suggesting that the biologic aggressiveness of breast cancer relates to the abnormal function of a limited number of genes (oncogenes). Furthermore, the abnormal function of these genes is thought to be reflected in certain properties of the breast cancer cell[17]. These cellular characteristics are called risk factors and correlate with the prognosis of breast cancer (see chapter 11).

Major risk factors. The following factors constitute major risk: tumor size; lymph node status; ER/PgR; tumor grade—HG, NG, MG: nuclear morphometry; DNA histogram, consisting of the S-phase fraction and DNA content (ploidy)—aneuploid versus diploid.

Minor risk factors. Microscopic adverse risk factors include foci of tumor necrosis, absence of microcalcifications, vascular invasion, lymphatic invasion, and infiltrative tumor border.

Computer programs. Some computer programs have recently been developed. Michael Retsky and colleagues[18] have devised a program that simulates the clinical behavior of breast cancer. The computer accepts the following clinical data: (1) size of the breast cancer, (2) number of positive axillary lymph nodes, (3) DNA content of the tumor, and (4) the treatment plan.

Recently Retsky and associates reported that this computer program was able to predict the disease-free survival of over 6,000 patients with an accuracy of 96 percent to 97 percent. This patient computerized prognosis analysis is now available for individual patients by contacting Michael Retsky, Ph.D, P.O. Box 7150, University of Colorado, Boulder, Colorado 80933-7150. See also the Appendix, section 5, for more information about this computer program.

When considered individually, these risk factors are each modest predictors of clinical behavior. However, when combinations of two or more unfavorable risk factors are considered together, they are powerful predictors of prognosis. The presence of two or more major adverse risk factors found in the plaintiff's breast cancer would suggest that the cancer had a growth rate two to three times faster than the average breast cancer, and that the tumor was a more aggressive breast cancer and had a greater potential to metastasize than the average breast cancer. Finding one or more adverse microscopic risk factors would lend support to this contention.

WHAT DO OTHERS SAY ABOUT OUR ABILITY TO IDENTIFY THE AGGRESSIVE BREAST CANCER?

Historically only node-positive women with breast cancer have received postoperative adjuvant chemotherapy. Node-negative women were thought to have an excellent prognosis, and postoperative adjuvant chemotherapy was not deemed necessary. Now we realize that 30 percent of node-negative women have aggressive breast cancer from which they will ultimately die. *Important Advances in Oncology 1989* contains an excellent article by Bonadonna and Valgussa that addresses this problem. The following is quoted from this article[19]:

. . . many prognostic indicators are now available to predict early relapse and short term survival in node negative breast cancer. In addition to negative hormone receptor status cell, proliferation activity—either expressed as high labeling index or high percent S-phase cells—should now be taken into consideration. Histopathologic evidence of undifferentiated (grade III) neoplastic cells and aneuploidy can be also added to the list of unfavorable prognostic parameters to improve patient selection. It should be stressed that we do not yet know the precise interrelationship of the unfavorable prognostic discriminants, and thus cannot determine how [many and which indicators will be necessary to accurately identify the aggressive breast cancer]. . . . Each of the above mentioned prognostic factors requires further study to convince clinicians that the new biologic findings can further improve treatment selection.

The authors then go on to say:

We suggest that clinicians seriously consider adjuvant therapy in node-negative breast cancer when there are at least two unfavorable prognostic indicators, such as grade III tumor and negative hormone receptors—particularly when both ER and PgR are absent. In hospitals where more sophisticated diagnostic facilities are available, the additional evidence of aneuploidy in the resected specimen, or of increased tumor cell proliferation activity by either thymidine-labeling or flow cytometry, should further alert physicians that the patient is at high risk [for the development of] micrometastatic disease. . . .

146

Clearly, then, the oncologists will now be doing the very thing we have been recommending: attempting to determine the aggressiveness of the breast cancer immediately following surgery. We, on the other hand, will be determining the aggressiveness of the tumor after it has recurred. The latter evaluation should be more accurate since we will be dealing with a group of cancers whose clinical behavior has indicated that they, as a group, are quite aggressive.

PROBLEMS OF INTERPRETATION OF RISK FACTORS

There is some overlapping of most risk factors. For example: Rapidly growing tumors tend to be ER − but a few will be ER +. Also, slow growing tumors tends to be ER + but a few will be ER −. Therefore, physicians will encounter an occasional breast tumor with conflicting risk factors, If a tumor is found with one favorable and two or three unfavorable risk factors, the physician should ignore the favorable factor.

THE RELATION OF GROWTH RATE AND AGGRESSIVENESS TO THE THRESHOLD SIZE

The growth rate and aggressiveness of a breast cancer have no effect on its threshold size. However, in the interval between screening examinations the rapidly growing aggressive cancer can attain a much larger size than the average breast cancer. Therefore, rapidly growing aggressive tumors may be quite large when first detected.

THE DOUBLING TIME DEFENSE: TO USE OR NOT TO USE

The growth rate of breast cancer is usually measured in doubling times, that is, the length of time required for a tumor to double the number of cancer cells in the tumor. For example:

Net Cell Doubling	Cancer Cells in the Tumor (Approximate)
10	1,000
20	1,000,000
30	1 billion
40	1 trillion

Since there are only about 11 trillion cells in the human body, the presence of 1 trillion cancer cells usually results in death for the patient. In the past the growth of breast cancer was thought to be exponential. Exponential growth is characterized by a constant rate of growth throughout the life of the tumor. Thus the doubling time would remain constant. It was thought that if we knew the size of the primary tumor and/or the metastasis plus the doubling time (commonly considered to be 100 days), we could extrapolate backwards and determine when the primary tumor and/or the metastasis originated. Unfortunately, the growth of breast cancer is not exponential but rather Gompertzian. Gompertzian growth is described as constantly decelerating throughout the life of the tumor. As the tumor increases in size, the cancer cells farthest from the capillary blood supply have difficulty obtaining oxygen, and the growth rate of the tumor slows. The problem is further complicated by the recent observation that there may be two to five plateaus in the life cycle of a cancer during which there is little or no growth[18]. Between these plateaus the growth is thought to be Gompertzian. Spratt[20] has stated that ''. . . attempts to extrapolate the growth curve beyond the extent of the observed data are subject to serious error.'' Extrapolating backwards with exponential doubling times in children with cancer has in some cases determined that the tumor originated several years before the child was born!

A Possible Exception

If, for example, the doubling time of a metastasis could be determined from serial measurements of the lesion in roentgenogram, it might be possible to extrapolate backwards and obtain a *rough approximation* of the size of the tumor 12 months previously.

A FINAL WORD

At the conclusion of the trial the jury should understand and be able to define the terms *threshold size* and *subthreshold size*, in addition to understanding the following facts:

- That all breast cancers have a threshold size.

That there is a wide variation in the threshold size of breast cancer.

- That it is impossible for a subthreshold breast cancer to be detected by any currently available diagnostic modality.
- That a dense breast increases the threshold size of breast cancer.
- That there is a small subset of breast cancers that spread systemically early in their life cycles long before they can be detected by any currently available diagnostic modality. As a result this group of cancers has great lethal potential.

Finally, this fact should be understood fully by the jury: The combination of a dense breast + a rapidly growing aggressive breast cancer = a potentially lethal situation. It constitutes a situation that is entirely beyond the control of the physician and, therefore, should not be the basis for a malpractice suit.

REFERENCES

1. Donegan WL. Staging and primary treatment. In *Cancer of the Breast*, 3rd ed. WB Saunders, 1988, pp. 336–402.
2. McKinnon NE. Cancer mortality: the failure to control through case finding programs. *S.G.O.* 94:173–178, 1952.
3. Bailer J III and Smith EM. Progress against cancer. *N Eng J Med* 314:1226–1232, 1986.
4. Skrabanek, P. False premises and false promises of breast cancer screening. *The Lancet*, August 10, 1985, pp. 316–320.
5. Editor. Science and the citizen. *Scientific American* 256:25, June 1987.
6. *Cancer Facts and Figures—1989*, American Cancer Society, 1989 p. 5.
7. *Cancer Facts and Figures—1989*, American Cancer Society, 1989, p. 15.
8. Gesme D. Personal communication, May 1989.
9. Spratt JS, Donegan WL, and Greenberg R. Screening and follow-up. In *Cancer of the Breast*, 3rd ed. Donegan and Spratt, eds. WB Saunders, 1988, pp. 558–590.
10. Koscielny S, et al. Breast Cancer: relationship between size of the primary tumor and the probability of metastatic dissemination. *Br J Cancer* 49:709–715, 1984.

11. Carter C, et al. Relation of tumor size, lymph node status, and survival in 24,700 breast cancer cases. *Cancer* 63:181–187 1989.

12. Tinnemans JGM, et al. Treatment and survival of female patients with nonpalpable breast carcinoma. *Ann Surg* 209(2):249–253, 1989

13. Spratt J and Spratt JS. Growth rates and cytokinetics of breast cancer. Lecture presented at the University of Heidelberg, October 1986. Personal communication.

14. Donegan, W. Diagnosis. In *Cancer of the Breast*, 3rd ed. Donegan and Spratt, eds. WB Saunders, 1988, pp. 125–166.

15. Fisher E. The impact of pathology on the biologic, diagnostic prognostic, and therapeutic considerations in breast cancer. *Surg Clin N Am* 64(6):1073–1093, 1984.

16. Fallenius A, et al. Predictive value of nuclear DNA content in breast cancer in relation to clinical and morphological factors. *Cancer* 62:521–530, 1988.

17. Hedley DW, et al. Association of DNA index and S-phase fraction with prognosis of nodes positive early breast cancer. *Cancer Research* 47:1–7, 1987.

18. Retsky M, et al. Prospective computerized simulation of breast cancer: comparison of computer predictions with nine sets of biological and clinical data. *Cancer Research* 47:4982–4987, 1987.

19. Bonadonna G and Valgussa P. Role of chemotherapy in Stage I breast cancer. In *Important Advances in Oncology—1989*. Devita, Hellman, and Rosenberg, eds. JP Lippincott, 1989, pp. 151–160.

20. Spratt JS and Spratt JA. Growth rates of cancer of the breast. In *Cancer of the Breast*, 3rd ed. Donegan and Spratt, eds. WB Saunders, 1988, p. 300.

19

ADDENDUM

Cellular biologists continue to identify new molecular factors that correlate with the aggressiveness of breast cancer[1]. Some seem quite promising and I predict that several will eventually prove quite useful to the medical malpractice defense attorney. A partial list would include:

Ki-67. A monoclonal antibody that binds to nuclear antigen present in cycling cells but not in resting cells. Ki-67 measures the proliferation rate of breast cancer and is said to be more accurate than a mitotic index established by counting the number of mitotic figures in 10 high power fields of an ordinary light microscope. This is important since there is a powerful correlation between the proliferation rate and the aggressiveness and metastatic potential of breast cancer. Not commonly used at present but should become available for the examination of fixed breast cancer tissue in the near future[2–4].

Cathepsin-D. A protease said to enhance the invasiveness of breast cancer[5]. Cathepsin-D sounds most promising but unfortunately it cannot be identified and measured in fixed breast cancer tissues at the present time[6].

Haptoglobin related protein [7]. I have found only one preliminary report but this sounded interesting. I understand reference laboratories are having difficulty gearing up for the processing of cancer tissue for this protein since the technique for analysis has been patented. It may not be available for some time.

Epidermal growth factor receptor [EGFR] [8]. Sainsbury found EGFR to be a powerful predictor of the lethal potential of breast

151

cancer, especially in lymph node negative cancers. His technique for the determination of the EGFR requires fresh tumor tissue[9]. Some laboratories are attempting to measure EGFR with immunocytochemical assays from fixed tissue but as yet they have been unsuccessful. It is hoped that this will become possible in the not too distant future.

C-erb B-2 protein (also known as **HER 2/neu**)[10]. The protein expression of the c-erb B-2 oncogene has been found to correlate with the prognosis of lymph node positive breast cancer. Increased expression of the protein for c-erb B-2 protein in the breast cancer of a woman with lymph node metastasis at the time of surgery would suggest that the cancer is unusually aggressive. C- erb B-2 can be determined from fixed tissue by immunocytochemical assay.

THESE NEW MOLECULAR FACTORS PRESENT SEVERAL PROBLEMS

1. Some require fresh or fresh-frozen tumor tissue, which is almost never available in the malpractice setting.
2. Some will ultimately prove to be more useful than others.
3. Many have undergone only preliminary clinical evaluation regarding their prognostic predictive ability. The significance of a positive test may, therefore, be questioned until more data are available. However, such data are rapidly becoming available.

RECOMMENDATIONS

If you should elect to explore the availability of one or more of these new molecular prognostic variables, do the following:

1. Contact a well-established and reliable reference laboratory such as the Nichols Institute or Cytometrics.

> Nichols Institute
> Worldway Postal Center
> P.O. Box 92797
> Los Angeles, CA 90009-2797

> Cytometrics, Inc.
> 11575 Sorrento Valley Road
> San Diego, CA 92121

They will be able to tell you which molecular risk factors can be identified and measured in fixed cancer tissue that has been embedded in paraffin blocks.

2. They should supply you with the values of the ''cutoff'' of high vs. low concentrations for the particular molecular risk factor under consideration.

3. They may be able to supply you with a list of references and review articles that discuss the clinical significance and limitations of these new molecular risk factors.

Which procedures can be performed from paraffin-embedded tissue? Present status, January, 1990

Nichols Institute
ER and PgR
DNA (ploidy and S-phase)

Cytometrics, Inc.
ER and PgR
DNA (ploidy and S-phase)
C-erb B-2 (also known as HER-2/neu)
Ki-67 monoclonal antibody. The proliferation rate of breast cancer is determined with the aid of a flow cytometer. I have been told that it may soon be possible to measure the growth rate of breast cancer in fixed sections of breast cancer using an image analyzer.
EGF-R. An immunocytochemical assay is in the development phase but as yet is not ready for clinical use. It may be available in the near future.

I am certain there are other excellent reference laboratories with which I am not familiar. When selecting a reference laboratory, try to select one with a staff of research scientists. Ask your expert witness to help you make the selection.

AGE AS A PROGNOSTIC RISK FACTOR

Pozner, et al.[11] found age to be a significant independent indicator of disease-free survival (DFS) in women with lymph node negative breast cancer. They reported that node negative women between the ages of 50 and 59 years had the highest 5-year DFS (89%). Younger women with lymph node negative disease had much poorer 5-year DFS. For example:

Women <50 years: 5-year DFS was 12% less than middle-aged women (50–59 years).

Women <40 years: 5-year DFS was 24% less than middle-aged women (50–59 years).

Therefore, when determining the aggressiveness of a lymph node negative breast cancer add age (if less than 50 years) to your combination of adverse risk factors. Age, in this study, was not found to be a significant prognostic risk factor in lymph node positive women.

REFERENCES

1. Abstracts #122–149. *Breast Cancer Research and Treatment* 14(1): 163–170, October 1989.
2. Bachus SS, et al. Biologic grading of breast cancer using antibodies to proliferating cells and other markers. *Am J. Path* 135(5): 783–792, 1989.
3. Hanna W, et al. Correlation of receptor status measured by the ERICA and Ki-67 growth fraction in human breast cancer. Abstract #122, *Breast Cancer Research and Treatment* 14(1): 163, October 1989.
4. Bonetti F, et al. Replicative fraction in breast carcinoma, an immunohistochemical study of 236 cases. Abstract #124, *Breast Cancer Research and Treatment* 14(1): 163, October 1989.
5. Spyratos F, et al. Cathepsin D: An independent prognostic factor for metastasis of breast cancer. *The Lancet*, November 11, 1989, pp. 1115–1118.
6. Rochefort, H. Personal communication. December 9, 1989.
7. Kuhajda FP, et al. Haptoglobin-related protein (Hpr) epitopes in breast cancer as a predictor of recurrence of the disease. *N Engl J Med* 321(10): 636–641, 1989.
8. Sainsbury JR, et al. Epidermal growth factor receptor status as predictor of early recurrence and death from breast cancer. *The Lancet*, June 20, 1987, p. 1389–1402.
9. Sainsbury JR. Personal communication. December 9, 1989.
10. Murayama Y, et al. Association of elevated expression of the c-erb B-2 protein with spread of breast cancer. Abstract #140, *Breast Cancer Research and Treatment* 14(1): 167, October 1989.
11. Pozner J, et al. Age as an independent prognostic indicator in breast carcinoma. Abstract #137 *Breast Cancer Research and Treatment* 14(10): 167, October 1989.

APPENDIX: DETERMINATION OF THE MALIGNANT POTENTIAL OF THE PLAINTIFF'S BREAST CANCER

1. EVALUATING THE ESTROGEN (ER) AND PROGESTERONE RECEPTOR (PgR) REPORTS

ER + /PgR + (41 percent of breast cancers)[1]

A positive estrogen receptor and a positive progesterone receptor (ER + /PgR +) have proven to be excellent predictors of a slower growing cancer with a better than average prognosis. If the plaintiff's breast cancer was ER + /PgR + , you will have difficulty proving that her cancer was growing more rapidly than the average breast cancer. There may well be small subsets of ER + / PgR + tumors that are quite aggressive, and these tumors might be identified by a diploid DNA and a high S-phase fraction or a DNA content that is aneuploid. However, at this time, it

155

may be difficult to identify this subset of breast cancers. Many centers are beginning to perform flow cytometry and hormone assays on all breast cancers, and in the near future we may be able to recognize this group of tumors.

ER + /PgR – (30 percent of breast cancers)[1]

The synthesis of the progesterone receptor is thought to be dependent upon the presence of a functioning estrogen receptor. Therefore, the absence of the progesterone receptor suggests that the estrogen recptor is either absent or nonfunctioning. Thus, an ER + /PgR – tumor contains a nonfunctioning or poorly functioning estrogen receptor. Actually, the five-year disease-free survival of ER + /Pgr – tumors is only marginally better (about 9 percent) than the five-year disease-free survival of ER – /PgR – tumors. Furthermore, in a large series of breast cancers the PgR was a significant predictor of a prolonged disease-free survival while the ER was not[2]. Thus, in a large series of breast cancers, knowing the status of the ER did not add to the predictive value of the PgR. Others have found that the concentration of the PgR is inversely related to the potential for metastases.

Therefore, when confronted with an ER + /PgR – tumor, employ the PgR status for your prediction. Ignore the ER status since it is nonfunctional. Consider the tumor to be ER – /PgR – .

ER – /PgR + (2 percent of patients + / –)[1]

In this situation the ER is falsely negative. Consider the tumor to be ER + /PgR + .

ER – /PgR – (27 percent of patients + / –)[1]

This group will be the easiest one with which to work. All agree that these tumors grow more rapidly and are more aggressive than ER + /PgR + tumors that constitute about 40 percent of all breast cancers. The risk of dying within five years is about two times greater when the tumor is ER – /PgR – versus an ER + /PgR + tumor. The following will tell you more about the predictive value of the hormone receptors.

ER/PgR and Nuclear Grade as Predictors of Outcome When Used in Combinations[3].

Fisher and associates[3] studied a large group of postoperative breast cancer patients who received adjuvant chemotherapy. They reported that the estrogen receptor (ER), progesterone receptor (PgR), and nuclear grade were each of modest and equal value as predictors of outcome when used singularly. When used in combination, however, they were powerful predictors of outcome. Table A1–1 summarizes Fisher's findings. Again, we note that although individual risk factors are predictive of outcome, combinations of unfavorable risk factors are more powerful predictors of an increased risk of dying from breast cancer.

Thus, if you have found:

One unfavorable risk factor.....................Risk dying/5 years + 10%
Two unfavorable risk factors.............Risk dying/5 years + 27% (2X)
Three unfavorable risk factors........Risk dying/5 years + 35% (2.5X)

If you have discovered two or three unfavorable risk factors, you have produced powerful evidence that the plaintiff's breast cancer was growing more rapidly and was more aggressive than the average breast cancer. That is, it was more aggressive than the 40 percent of breast tumors that are ER + /PgR + .

TABLE A1-1. SUMMARIZES FISHER'S FINDINGS

	RISK OF DYING IN FIVE YEARS
All three factors favorable	
ER above 10 f/mols)	
PgR above 10 f/mols)	23%
Nuclear grade good)	
One factor unfavorable	27 to 33%
Two factors unfavorable	50%
All factors unfavorable	
ER 0-9 f/mol)	
PgR 0-9 f/mol)	58%
Nuclear grade poor)	

The ER/PgR Status as a Predictor of the Rate of Cell Division[4]

Moran and associates[4] have demonstrated an interesting correlation between the ER/PgR status and the rate of cell division as expressed by the S-phase fraction of the DNA (determined by flow cytometry). It is interesting that the rate of cell division of ER+/PgR− and ER−/PgR− tumors is almost twice as great as the rate of cell division of ER+/Pgr+ tumors.

	Mean (%) S-phase Fraction	
ER+/PgR+	11%	The % of tumor
ER+/pgR−	19%	cells that are
ER−/PgR−	20%	actively dividing

Modified from Moran et al.[4].

Since about 27 percent of breast cancers are ER−/PgR− and 30 percent are ER+/PgR−, about 57 percent of breast cancer will have a high proliferation rate and will be growing about twice as fast as the ER+/PgR+ tumors.

PgR Is a More Powerful Predictor of Outcome Than Is the ER

Clark and colleagues[2] agree that although the absence of the estrogen receptor and the progesterone receptor both predict a shorter disease-free interval or survival rate, the PgR is a more significant predictor of disease-free interval than is the ER. The authors defined a negative receptor as:

ER—less than 3 fmol. of specific binding sites of the estrogen receptor per milligram of cytosol protein.
PgR—less than 5 fmol. of specific binding sites of the progesterone per milligram of cytosol protein.
Note—fmol. is an abbreviation for *femto,* a Danish word that means 15, and *mole,* or molecular weight. When femto is used as a unit of measurement, it indicates 10^{-15} or one quadrillion, in this case, one-quadrillionth of the molecular weight of the estrogen or progesterone receptor per milligram of cytosol protein.

Caveat

The medical literature regarding the prognostic predictive

value of the hormone receptors is confusing and difficult to interpret. There are a number of reasons for this[5]: (1) the number of women in many series is quite small; (2) the periods of observation often are quite short; and (3) receptor assay values vary from laboratory to laboratory.

After careful "sifting out" of the evidence, I think we can state that the available evidence supports the following conclusions:

1. ER − /PgR − tumors grow faster than ER + /Pgr + tumors.

2. The disease-free survival of ER + tumors is significantly higher than ER− tumors at 12 and 24 months.

3. Sometime after 36 months[6] the survival curves of the ER+ and the ER− women tend to merge. At the end of five years the survival advantage of the ER+ woman is about 10 percent greater than the ER − woman[7].

4. Although the prognostic predictive power of an unfavorable estrogen or progesterone receptor is only modest when used alone, when combined with two or more other unfavorable risk factors, their predictive value is much greater.

2. HISTOLOGIC FEATURES AS INDICATORS OF GROWTH RATE AND LETHALITY

Consult Your Pathologist.

Obtain copies of the articles by Bloom[8], Parl[9], and Russo[10]. Ask the pathologist to read these articles and this section of this book before he or she grades the plaintiff's breast cancer.

Histologic Grading (Pathologic Grade)

Table A2–1 summarizes the criteria used for the pathologic grading of tumors according to the histologic features found in the breast cancer.

Investigators familiar with the grading of breast cancer agree that the histologic grade (HG), the nuclear grade (NG), and the mitotic grade (MG) are each significant predictors of tumor recurrence and death. Some, however, have found the nuclear grade (NG) to be more accurate. Russo[10] has reported:

159

TABLE A2–1. CRITERIA USED FOR GRADING OF TUMORS

HISTOLOGIC GRADE		NUCLEAR GRADE	MITOTIC GRADE
Grade I (good)	Well-developed tubules	Most differentiated, uniform size, shape, and chromatin staining	0–10/10 hpf.*
Grade II (moderate)	Moderate tubule formation	Moderate variation in size and shape	11–20/10 hpf.*
Grade III (poor) or (high)	Slight to no differentiation of tubules. Cells in sheets.	Marked immaturity with great variation in size	+21/10 hpf.*

*hpf = high power field of ordinary light microscope.
Source: Modifed from Russo [10].

48-Month Disease-Free Survival of Breast Cancer for Lymph Node-Negative Patients
Mitotic Grade I...92%
Mitotic Grades II & III 76%

Russo[10] also found histologic Grades I and II, nuclear Grades I and II, and mitotic Grades II and III to have similar survival rates. Therefore, when employing the histologic features of a tumor to determine the risk of recurrence, consider the tumor grades with similar survival rates as a unit. For example:

HG I & II	vs.	HG III
NG I & II	vs.	NG III
MG I	vs.	MG II & III

Combinations Are Important

Parl[9] found combinations of adverse risk factors (table A2–2) to be predictors of an increased risk of death from breast cancer.

Parl's data clearly demonstrate that each histologic risk

factor predicts a significant increase in the risk of dying from breast cancer. However, when used in combinations, they are more powerful predictors of an increased risk of death from breast cancer.

Others have also stressed the increased predictive power of combinations of adverse risk factors. Russo[10] employed combinations of MG, lymph node status, ER, and tumor size. Each of these risk factors was thought to identify high risk women not identified by the other three. When two or three of these risk factors agreed, the risk of recurrence was extremely high.

Fisher and associates[3] found that combinations of ER, PgR, and nuclear grade were powerful predictors of the survival of breast cancer (see Appendix, section 1).

The Classic Article of Bloom[8]

The classic article of Bloom in 1950 clearly demonstrated the prognostic value of the histologic features of breast cancer. His conclusions, published 40 years ago, are still valid today. He also tells us the number of patients in each category (see table A2-3).

The distribution of the patients in the Russo and associates[10] series of 646 women was similar to Bloom's series except that Russo had fewer patients in mitotic Grades II and III (see table A2-4).

Tables A2-2 and A2-3 tell us the frequency of Grades I, II, and III in over 1,000 breast cancer patients. This will give us some idea of how often we can expect a patient to fall into one of these grades.

Evaluating the Mitotic Grade (mitotic frequency or index)

The significance of the frequency of mitotic figures in breast cancer has been clouded by the conflicting data in the literature. There are several reasons for this:

1. The degree of differentiation (maturity) of the cancer cells within a breast cancer often is not uniform. Not uncommonly, there will be areas within the tumor that are much less differentiated (more immature). These areas are more rapidly growing. Since the prognosis of the breast cancer will be deter-

TABLE A2–2. HISTOLOGIC FACTORS AND INCREASED RISK OF DYING FROM INFILTRATING DUCT CELL CANCER OF THE BREAST (70 CASES)

HISTOLOGIC RISK FACTOR	FREQUENCY	INCREASE RISK OF DYING IN 10 YEARS
High Nuclear Grade	17/70	2x
Frequent Mitotic Figures	11/70	4x
High Histologic Grade	37/70	7x
High Histologic Grade and Frequent Mitotic Figures	9/70	13x
High Histologic Grade and High Nuclear Grade	13/70	20x

Source: Modified from Parl [9].

TABLE A2–3. INDIVIDUAL GRADING FACTORS AND SURVIVAL

FACTOR	DEGREE	# CASES	FIVE YR. SURVIVAL
Tubule Formation	Well marked	105	73%
	Moderate	256	42%
	Slight or nil	109	39%
Variation of nuclei	Slight	87	72%
	Moderate	225	58%
	Marked	158	29%
Mitotic figures	Very few or nil	73	86%
	Moderate	231	52%
	Marked	166	27%

Source: Modified from Bloom [8].

TABLE A2-4. DISTRIBUTION OF PATIENTS IN RUSSO ET AL. SERIES [11] (646 patients)

	I	II	III
HG	7	62	577
NG	21	389	236
MG	496	79	71

Source: Modified from Russo et al. [10].

mined by the behavior of the cancer cells within these undifferentiated regions, count the number of mitoses in these areas. *Do not take counts in average or random areas. This will result in a falsely low mitotic index.*

2. Usually the number of cells in mitosis in 10 high power fields are counted. Unfortunately, the area encompassed by 10 high power fields varies depending upon the microscope and the optical system used for the count. For this reason, some are counting the number of mitotic figures per square millimeter rather than 10 high power fields.

3. The number of tumor cells in a high power field will vary according to the ratio of cancer cells and benign stroma. Try to count in areas with little benign stroma.

4. The count should include *all* of the tumor cells in *any phase* of mitosis.

5. When tumor cells degenerate, the nucleus may become shrunken (pyknosis) or the nucleus may rupture, extruding its chromatin from the cell (karyorrhexis). The inexperienced observer may mistake these degenerating nuclei for mitotic figures. Experienced observers state that this is not a problem.

Technique for Obtaining an Accurate Mitotic Index
As described by Russo and associates[10], the technique for obtaining an accurate mitotic index is as follows:

1. Search the slide under low power to find the most undifferentiated areas of the tumor. Count in these areas.

2. Use a Zeiss or American Optics microscope.

3. Count 10 40x fields using a 10x ocular.

4. Count the total number of cells in *any phase* of mitosis.

If you have difficulty in obtaining a proper pathologic grade and/or a mitotic index, consider sending the slides to someone who has done research in this area.

What Is a Typical Mitotic Count?
McDivitt and colleagues[11] proposed a classification of breast cancer based on kinetic information. They studied 106 consecutive cases of breast cancer. The histology of the cancers varied as indicated below:

Ordinary infiltrative duct cell carcinoma.............................73.8%
Atypical medullary adenocarcinoma...................................8.3%
Lobular adenocarcinoma 5.3%
Intraductal adenocarcinoma...4.1%
Medullary adenocarcinoma..3.6%
Colloid adenocarcinoma..1.2%

For the mitotic count, 10 contiguous high power fields were counted employing an ordinary light microscope using the 20x objective[11].

# of mitoses per 10 high power fields.............................0 to 106
Mean (average) 13
Median 7.5

Typical Mitotic Counts in Breast Cancer

Kuhns[12] testified in a malpractice suit involving breast cancer and stated the following: The average number of mitotic figures is 0-4/10 hpf (high power field). The count is considered high if 5-15/10 hpf. He seldom finds more than 12-15/10 hpf.

Is Pathologic Grading Reliable?

All agree that the pathologic grading of tumors (HG, NG, and MG) correlates with prognosis. Nevertheless, some charge that the pathologic grading of breast cancers is subjective and that, in situations where the pathologist is unfamiliar with criteria for grading and/or he or she has little interest or experience in tumor grading, there may be considerable intraobserver and interobserver variation in the pathologic grading of breast cancers.

It is generally agreed, however, that pathologic grading performed by experienced observers is quite accurate. Bloom and Richardson[13] independently graded over 400 breast cancers with an interobservor agreement of over 90 percent.

Tips for Improving Accuracy of Grading

A few things can be suggested for improving accuracy in grading. First, help the pathologist obtain the material with which to become familiar with the strict criteria for pathologic grading. Second, use a standard technique for the mitotic count (see Russo[10]). Finally, encourage the pathologist to use the diameter of the red blood cell and lymphocyte when judging the size of a tumor cell and/or nucleus.

Tumor Grading

The recent literature continues to reinforce the value of tumor grading. Hanson[14] from the National Cancer Institute reported that the grading of breast cancer provides prognostic information in addition to that provided by stage (lymph node status and tumor size). He concluded that the grading of breast cancer can substantially improve the prediction of outcome that is predicted by lymph node status. This is additional support for the concept that combinations of risk factors are more predictive of outcome. Most investigators agree that expertise of tumor grading is not widespread since few pathologists have interest in this area[14,15]. Thus, if you plan to incorporate tumor grading in your defense, try to find a pathologist who has a special interest in this phase of pathology.

Lymph Node Status, Tumor Size, and Mitotic Index

Van Der Linden et al.[16] report that breast cancers containing more than 9 mitotic figures per 10 high power fields have a significantly increased risk of recurrence. For example, 90% of breast cancer patients with less than 9 mitoses per 10 high power fields are disease free at 49 months while only 60% of those with more than 9 mitoses per 10 high power fields are disease free at 49 months. The authors compared the prognostic accuracy of lymph node status, tumor size, and mitotic index versus lymph node status alone. After five years the combination of lymph node status, tumor size, and mitotic index provided more accurate information regarding prognosis for 20% of the patients than did lymph node status alone[16].

Lymph Node Status, Tumor Size, and Tumor Grade

In England, Blamey[17], Haybittle et al.[18], and Todd et al.[19] have found that lymph node status, tumor size, and tumor grade (Nottingham Index) is a much more powerful predictor of outcome than lymph node status alone. Once again we have support for the value of combinations of risk factors. Using the Nottingham Index, Todd et al.[19] were able to divide 21% of their patients into two groups:

Low-risk group—88% survived for 8 years
High-risk group—7% survived for 8 years

The remaining 79% of their patients could be divided into three groups[19].

Low-risk group—78% survived for 8 years
Intermediate group—60% survived for 8 years
High-risk group—30% survived for 8 years

The Nottingham Index can, if properly used, easily identify women whose cancers are more aggressive than the average. For additional information about the Nottingham Index, contact *J. H. Todd, City Hospital, Nottingham NG5, UK.*

3. THE SIGNIFICANCE OF COMBINATIONS OF ADVERSE RISK FACTORS

A simple diagram clearly illustrates the power of combining risk factors. Thus:

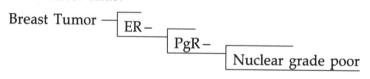

Risk factors are either favorable or unfavorable. Consider the estrogen receptor (ER). An ER + status is a favorable risk factor since these tumors grow more slowly than ER − tumors. On the other hand, an ER − status is an unfavorable risk factor since these tumors tend to grow more rapidly.

When we eliminate the ER + tumors we have excluded about 50 percent of the breast cancers (all slower growing).

Next, consider the progesterone receptor (PgR). A few

ER– tumors will be PgR+. Again, this group of tumors with a favorable risk will be excluded.

Now, consider nuclear grade. Some tumors will have a good nuclear grade and these, too, will be excluded.

Each time we add an unfavorable risk factor to our combination, we have eliminated a group of tumors with a favorable risk factor. Therefore, a group of tumors with two, three, or more unfavorable risk factors is strongly predictive of an increased risk of dying from breast cancer.

Since each unfavorable risk factor identifies a few high-risk patients not recognized by the other adverse risk factors, it is important to continue our search for additional unfavorable risk factors.

4. MICROSCOPIC ADVERSE RISK FACTORS

The following are all microscopic adverse risk factors for which prognostic predictive value has been documented in the literature: absence of microscopic calcifications within the tumor, infiltrative tumor borders, vascular invasion within the tumor, tumor emboli within the blood vessels in the breast tissue surrounding the tumor, lymphatic invasion or tumor emboli within the tumor, lymphatic invasion or tumor emboli in the breast tissue surrounding the tumor, perineural lymphatic invasion, and focal areas of necrosis within the tumor.

Were any adverse microscopic risk factors found in the plaintiff's breast cancer? If so, add them to your list of combinations of unfavorable risk factors since they can be important. Some may consider these findings to be of little predictive value. Many pathologists do not make a special effort to search for these items and, as a result, it is difficult to obtain adequate numbers of some of these factors with which to conduct accurate studies. *Nevertheless, none are favorable findings since they are not seen in slow-growing indolent tumors.* Recent studies have shown them to be of significant predictive value. Actually, these microscopic observations have captured and preserved one small step in the inexorable process of the local invasion and metastasis of a virulent breast cancer. If one or more of these findings can be added to previously assembled combinations of two or more adverse risk factors, convincing evidence will be supplied that the plaintiff's breast cancer was indeed more invasive than the average breast cancer.

Heuser and colleagues[20] found that the absence of calcifications within the tumor and the presence of lymphatic invasion around the periphery of the tumor were significantly associated with the development of early metastases.

Gilchrist[21] studied 774 women who had been treated with surgery and chemotherapy for node-positive breast cancer. He reported that the finding of clusters of necrotic tumor cells within the tissue specimens predicted an early recurrence of the breast cancer.

Blamey and associates[22] found that tumors containing areas of vascular invasion were more likely to recur locally.

Fischer and associates[23] studied the pathology of 1,000 invasive breast cancers from the National Surgical Adjuvant Breast Project (protocol#4). The pathologic examination was initially performed by the participating medical centers. throughout the country. Paraffin blocks of tumor tissue were also sent to the national headquarters for additional study. All questionable lesions were independently judged by two referees and disagreements settled by consensus. Conclusions from this most impressive study are described below.

Circumscribed versus infiltrative, irregular stellate borders. The lack of a circumscribed tumor border was associated with an increase in the short-term treatment failure at 18 and 24 months.

Degree of tumor necrosis. Two-thirds of tumors exhibited some tumor necrosis. Tumors with moderate and marked tumor necrosis demonstrated a higher degree of anaplasia.

Lymphatic invasion. Lymphatic invasion within the tumor and in the quadrants of the breast were associated with an increase in the risk of short-term treatment failure at 18 and 24 months.

Perineural lymphatic invasion. This was observed in 27.8 percent of breast cancers, and was associated with lymphatic inva-

sion, nipple involvement, axillary metastases, and an increase
in short-term treatment failure.

Blood vessel invasion. Blood vessel invasion was observed in
4.7 percent of the breast cancers and was associated with
marked tumor necrosis and increased axillary metastases. No
increase in short-term treatment failure was noted.

Nipple involvement. An increase in short-term treatment failure was noted.

Involvement of the skin over the tumor. An increase in short-
term treatment failure was noted.

Sinus histiocytosis. This was thought to indicate host immune
response. If sinus histiocytosis was absent, an increase in
short-term treatment failure was noted at 18 months.

5. NEW TESTS: FLOW CYTOMETRY

It has been known for over 100 years that nuclear abnormalities
are related to the risk of recurrence of cancer. It is not surprising, therefore, that recent studies reveal that the nuclear DNA
content provides reliable information regarding the malignant
potential of the breast cancer cell. DNA flow cytometry tells us
two important facts concerning the DNA of the breast cancer
cell[24,25]:

    1. The percentage of cancer cells whose DNA is in the
synthesis phase (S-phase) of cell division. The S-phase correlates well with the growth rate of the cancer, but at present its
usefulness is limited due to technical difficulties.

    2. The nuclear DNA content. When the DNA of the tumor
cell is stained and examined with a laser beam, the degree of
fluorescence of the nuclei tells us whether the amount of DNA
of the cancer cell is normal or near normal (diploid), less than
normal (hypodiploid), or greater than normal (hyperdiploid,
tetraploid, hypertetraploid, multiploid, etc.). Auer's[26] classification of the DNA is said to give the greatest predictive
power. It will be easier to understand this classification if we
understand the following:

Number of chromosomes in each human cell = 46.
Haploid = having the reduced number of chromosomes as in the
  sperm cell or the ovum (23 chromosomes).

Diploid = (twofold) having double the haploid number of chromosomes, that is, the normal number of chromosomes.

Tetraploid = (fourfold) having four haploid sets of chromosomes.

Aneuploid = (not well folded) having an uneven number of the multiple of the normal number of chromosomes.

The nuclear DNA content of the breast cancer cell provides a reliable and objective predictor of the malignant potential of breast cancer (see table A5–1). The analysis of the DNA content has become an important and useful tool in defining subsets of patients with high probability of short-term relapse. This will prove invaluable in selecting patients who will benefit from adjuvant therapy following surgery. *Defense should use this same technique to identify breast cancers whose adverse results may have been secondary to the malignant potential of the tumor rather than physician error.*

Hedley and colleagues[28] have demonstrated that the DNA content of breast cancer cells can be determined from archival paraffin-embedded tumor tissue as well as from fresh frozen tumor. Your pathologist should be able to locate a laboratory capable of performing this examination. If not, try Nichols Institute, Reference Laboratories, 26441 Via De Anaz, San Juan Capistrano, CA 92675, 1-800-LAB-TEST, 1-800-522-8378. Ask that they use the Auer classification of the DNA content.

Fallenius[27] also found evidence that aneuploidy occurs early in the neoplastic process and antedates the invasive stage of breast cancer. This lends credence to the concept of biologic predetermination.

The following definitions are used in interpreting the DNA histogram. As the degree of distortion of the DNA increases from hyperdiploid to hypotetraploid to tetraploid to hypertetraploid to multiploid, the aggressiveness of the tumor tends to increase. Some have found hypodiploid tumors to have an especially poor prognosis.

Diploid. Suggests the tumor is well differentiated and has a low risk of recurrence.

Diploid with a low S-phase. Node-negative tumors that are diploid and have a low S-phase (below 6.7 percent) have an

TABLE A5–1. THE PREDICTIVE VALUE OF THE NUCLEAR DNA CONTENT OF 227 CONSECUTIVE BREAST CANCER CASES: THE TEN YEAR RECURRENCE-FREE SURVIVAL

Axillary lymph nodes negative	
All patients	72%
DNA content (Auer's classification)	
Diploid (I)	95%
Tetraploid (II)	75%
Aneuploid (III & IV)	57%
Axillary lymph nodes positive	
All patients	45%
DNA content	
Diploid (I)	76%
Tetraploid (II)	45%
Aneuploid (III IV)	31%

Source: Modified from Fallenius et al. [27].

excellent prognosis. Ninety percent will live for 10 years[29].

Diploid with a high S-phase. Diploid tumors with a high S-phase (above 6.7 percent) have a five-year survival that is similar to an aneuploid tumor[29].

Aneuploid tumors. The three- to five-year recurrence for aneuploid tumors is about two or more times greater than a diploid tumor. This is true regardless of the S-phase. Meyer[30] stated that many studies indicated that the probabilities of relapse and death within three to five years is increased two or more times if the tumor is aneuploid rather than diploid.

Hyperdiploid tumors. Have a slightly higher recurrence rate than diploid tumors.

Hypodiploid tumors. Classified as aneuploid and have the same or even worse prognosis.

Tetraploid tumors. Classified as aneuploid and have the same prognosis? Check with your expert or laboratory.

Hypertetraploid tumors. Classified as aneuploid and have the same prognosis.

DNA Index

The DNA index is obtained by dividing the channel number of the aneuploid cells in the DNA histogram by the channel number of the diploid cells. The DNA index of diploid cells is arbitrarily set at 1.0. Thus, a tumor with a DNA index of 1.4 contains more DNA than the tumor with a DNA index of 1.2. A hypodiploid tumor has a DNA index which is less than 1.0. The DNA index correlates with prognosis. The greater the DNA index, the poorer the prognosis.

Caveat

Recent literature continues to support the concept that the DNA content of the tumor correlates with the clinical behavior of breast cancer, Experienced observors, however, suggest that caution should be used when evaluating the results of DNA flow cytometry.

S-Phase. It is generally agreed that it is not possible to determine the S-phase in about 20% of specimens. In addition, the S-phase of solid tumors such as breast cancer will vary significantly depending upon[31,32]:

1. The histology of the specimen (infiltrating duct cell, infiltrating lobular, medullary, etc.)
2. Type of specimen processed (frozen, paraffin block).
3. Method of preparing the specimen.
4. DNA staining.
5. Type of flow cytometer employed.
6. Computer software used.
7. Number of cells examined.
8. Number of benign stromal cells in the specimen.

As a result, it may be difficult to evaluate the S-phase value of an individual specimen. Clark and McQuire[32] and Hedley (33) and others, however, have found that by comparing a high with a low S-phase it is possible to obtain a valid prediction of clinical behavior in about two-thirds of the cases.

Ploidy. Most authors agree that aneuploidy is a modest predictor of an increased risk of treatment failure. Some[34], however, report that this is true only for the lymph-node-positive women. Others[29, 35–37] have found that aneuploidy predicts an increased risk of recurrence for the node-negative as well as the node-positive woman. It is possible that variations in technique may explain some of these differences.

It is obvious, therefore, that we cannot draw valid comparisons of the data from different investigators unless we know that they are employing similar methods for measuring S-phase and ploidy.

Combinations of S-phase and ploidy. Some authors report that combinations of S-phase and ploidy[29] or S-phase and DNA index[37] more accurately predict prognosis than ploidy alone. Clark et al.[29] performed DNA flow cytometric analysis of 395 women with node negative breast cancer. They determined the 6-year disease free survival of these 395 women by S-phase and ploidy status:

DNA Content	Number of patients	6 year disease-free survival
Diploid/low S-phase	112	88%
Diploid/high S-phase	15	56%
Aneuploid/with any S-phase	233	71%

Conclusion

Until this controversy has been settled and the procedures for the analysis of the DNA content has become standardized, try to minimize the variables. Do the following:

1. Select a medical witness who is thoroughly familiar with the technique of DNA flow cytometry, its limitations, and its clinical significance.

2. Ask your DNA expert to select the laboratory to which you will send the sample of breast tissue. It is important that your consultant be familiar with and have confidence in the accuracy of the S-phase and ploidy values of the tissue about which he or she is asked to render an opinion.

Computerized Simulation of the Clinical Behavior of Breast Cancer

Michael Retsky and his colleagues[38] at the University of Colorado have developed a computer program that accepts the following clinical data from the individual patient: tumor size, lymph node status, DNA content, and proposed treatment (surgery and chemotherapy).

The computer compares this information with data (obtained from some of the world's best medical literature) with 2,500 patients who have precisely the same clinical presentation. From this, the computer predicts the probability of the patient's being disease-free each year for 15 years.

This computer-generated prognosis system has been tested using archival data from 5,823 breast cancer patients from the University of Texas Health Science Center—San Antonio. The computer predicted the probability of each patient's being disease-free yearly for a period of 15 years, with an average error of only 4 percent. The archival data were obtained through the courtesy of Dr. G. Clark and Dr. W. McGuire. The system has also been tested against archival data from 564 patients from the University of Leiden, The Netherlands, with an average error of 3 percent. It is my understanding that Retsky and his colleagues are planning to add patient age and menopausal status, estrogen and progesterone receptor levels, tamoxifen therapy, and the number of lymph nodes examined to the computer model in the near future[39].

Dr. Retsky[39] tells me that he knows of only one criticism of his computer model. Those interested in a critical evaluation of this model should consult: L. Norton (A Gompertzian model of human breast cancer growth, *Cancer Research* 48:7076–7071, December 15, 1988) and the response by Michael Retsky (Letter to the editor, *Cancer Research*, forthcoming).

This computerized management system is now available for individual patients. For more information contact: Michael Retsky, Ph.D., P.O. Box 7150, Colorado Springs, CO 80933-7150.

6. NEW TESTS: NUCLEAR MORPHOMETRY

Nuclear morphometry is a seldom used procedure, but it is

said to be inexpensive and a good predictor of lethality. If you are having difficulty obtaining a nuclear grade and mitotic index of the plaintiff's cancer, you might consider corresponding with one of the investigators experienced with this technique. Nuclear morphometry is performed by obtaining a photomicrograph of the plaintiff's breast cancer. The image is greatly enlarged and then projected onto a special screen containing horizontal and vertical lines spaced at intervals of one micron. From this, the mean nuclear area and mitotic index can be easily calculated. The mitotic index is calculated by counting the number of sharply defined mitoses in 10 high power fields at a magnification of 400x using a 40x objective.

Baack and associates[40] found the mitotic index and the mean nuclear area as determined by nuclear morphometry to be powerful predictors of prognosis (see table A6-1) . The authors also studied the prognostic significance of nuclear grade and histologic grade[40].

The data in table A6-2 regarding nuclear grade and histologic grade confirm the data presented earlier by Parl.

Dr. Baack's address is: Jan P. Baack, M.D., PhD., Institute of Pathology, Free University, De Boelelaan 1117, 1007 MB, Amsterdam, The Netherlands.

Maehle and colleagues[41] also reported an excellent correlation between the mean nuclear area and the survival rate of breast cancer at ten years (see table A6-3).

Dr. Maehle's address is: Dr. B.O. Maehle, Department of Pathology, Haukeland Hospital, 5016 Bergen, Norway.

7. WHAT WAS THE HISTOLOGIC TYPE OF THE PLAINTIFF'S BREAST CANCER?

The histologic type of the plaintiff's breast cancer will only be of a little help (see table A7-1). If her tumor was an infiltrating duct cell or infiltrating lobular cell carcinoma, it was one of the 85 percent of breast cancers with the poorest survival rate. The other 15 percent have a much higher survival rate[42].

About one-third of invasive ductal carcinomas contain microscopic foci of areas resembling tubular, medullary, papillary, or mucinous differentiation. However, if the tumor is primarily infiltrating ductal carcinoma, the presence of these

TABLE A6–1. MITOTIC INDEX AND MEAN NUCLEAR AREA AS PREDICTORS OF PROGNOSIS

		% FIVE-YEAR SURVIVAL
Mitotic Index		
less than	10	88
	10–20	69
greater than	20	50
Mean Nuclear Area*		
less than	37 um²*	81
	37–53 um²	69
greater than	53 um²	57

*um² = square microns.
Source: Modified from Baack et al. [40].

TABLE A6–2. NUCLEAR GRADE AND HISTOLOGIC GRADE AS PREDICTORS OF PROGNOSIS

	% FIVE-YEAR SURVIVAL
Nuclear Grade	
Well differentiated	96
Moderately well differentiated	74
Poorly differentiated	66
Histologic grade	
Well differentiated	97
Moderately well differentiated	78
Poorly differentiated	55

Source: Modified from Baack et al. [40].

TABLE A6–3. CORRELATION BETWEEN MEAN NUCLEAR AREA AND SURVIVAL RATE

MEAN NUCLEAR AREA		% SURVIVAL AT TEN YEARS
Less than 44.8 um²*	(25% of patients)	50
44.8–71.4 um²	(50% of patients)	27
Greater than 71.4 um²	(25% of patients)	18

*um² = square microns.

Source: Modified from Maehle et al. [41].

TABLE A7-1. HISTOLOGIC TYPE OF BREAST CANCER AND THE RISK OF DYING IN TEN YEARS

HISTOLOGIC TYPE OF CARCINOMA	FREQUENCY	RISK OF DYING WITHIN TEN YEARS
Infiltrating duct cell	78.1%	53%
Infiltrating lobular cell	8.7%	58%
Infiltrating medullary	4.3%	32%
Infiltrating comedo	4.6%	23%
Infiltrating colloid	2.6%	28%
Infiltrating papillary	1.2%	35%
Tubular	rare	low
Adenocystic	rare	low

Source: Modified from McDivitt (42).

more favorable histologic types has no influence on the prognosis[43].

8. HAS THE PLAINTIFF DEVELOPED EVIDENCE OF SYSTEMIC BREAST CANCER?[44,45]

There are three large subgroups of breast cancers:

1. Forty percent + / – of women have slow-growing indolent cancers that almost never spread systemically.

2. Twenty percent + / – of women have breast cancers with an intermediate growth rate and a variable ability to metastasize.

3. Forty percent + / – of women have rapidly growing aggressive breast cancers that metastasize early and kill 25 percent of the women each year with or without treatment.

If the plaintiff has developed evidence of systemic breast cancer, she certainly does not belong to the 40 percent group of women with slow-growing indolent breast cancers that seldom metastasize. Our search for unfavorable risk factors should help us identify the malignant potential of the plaintiff's breast cancer.

9. NOTES FROM "THE CUTTING EDGE"

Anyone who has experience in the treatment of breast cancer can agree with Henderson[46] when he states "It is important to remember that most breast cancers—certainly more than

50%—die of a more indolent variety of the disease." He went on to say that we should be placing more emphasis on looking at such things as growth factors (and other agents and techniques) as they emerge from the laboratory. We do need help in identifying the woman who is destined to die from the indolent varient of breast cancer. Hopefully some of the methodologies from "the cutting edge" will prove useful.

Haptoglobin-Related Protein (Hpr) Predicts Recurrence of Breast Cancer

Kuhajda, Piantadosi, and Pasternack[47] recently reported that breast cancer cells whose cytoplasm contains a poorly understood glycoprotein, called a haptoglobin-related protein (Hpr), have significantly greater risk of treatment failure. Immunohistochemical analysis of routinely processed paraffin blocks of tumor tissue can be used to detect this unusual protein. Archival paraffin blocks of breast cancer tissue should be available for virtually all breast cancer patients.

The authors observed that Hpr-positive early breast cancers developed recurrent disease much sooner than Hpr-negative early breast cancer. For example, 40% of Hpr-positive early breast cancers developed recurrence within 2 years while 40% of Hpr-negative early breast cancers developed recurrence within 8 1/2 years[47].

In addition, the combination of Hpr reactivity (Hpr-positive) and the absence of the progesterone receptor (PgR-negative) was found to be a powerful predictor of clinical behavior of breast cancer. For example[47]:

Hpr and PgR receptor	% Recurrence at 8 years	Number of patients in study
Hpr + /PgR –	92%	11/12
Hpr + /PgR +	45%	5/12
Hrp – /PgR +	24%	6/25
Hpr – /PgR –	19%	3/16

This preliminary report of this small series suggests that the presence of the Hpr protein in the cytoplasm of the breast cancer cell may prove to be a reliable predictor of prognosis. Furthermore, there are indications that Hpr reactivity when combined with other adverse risk factors may prove to be an even more powerful discriminant of the risk of treatment failure.

Kuhajda et al.[47] also compared the Hpr reactivity of the primary tumors of a group of unselected breast cancers with the primary tumors of 14 women who had died of breast cancer. Of the unselected primary breast cancers, 39.5% were Hpr reactive while the Hpr reactivity of the primary tumors of women dying of breast cancer was twice as high (79%).

Lance Liotta from the National Cancer Institute stated (48) "we can see in the future there will be a number of these tests and they will all be incorporated into a panel of markers" to predict the likelihood of metastases. For reprints and information concerning the haptoglobin-related protein, contact Dr. F.P. Kuhajda, M.D., Department of Pathology, Johns Hopkins Hospital, 600 North Wolfe Street, Baltimore, MD, 21205.

Oncogenes

Recent literature continues to suggest that alterations in proto-oncogenes and/or oncogenes are somehow related to the progression and aggressiveness of breast cancer[47,49]. A number of oncogenes have been studied but thus far the oncogene HER-2/neu seems to one of the more promising[47,49,50]. In general, information from the study of oncogenes needs additional study before this data will be useful in the clinical setting. However, there may be a possible exception. If 10 mg of tumor tissue is available, the measurement of the protein product of the oncogene HER-2/neu from a lymph-node-positive tumor could be helpful. (Western blot technique)[50]. The discovery of the overproduction of the protein product of the oncogene HER-2/neu in a lymph-node-positive patient would suggest that you have identified a tumor that is more aggressive than the average lymph-node-positive breast cancer[49].

Growth Factors

Some tumor cells not only secrete growth factors but respond to the growth factors that they secrete as well as to other growth factors. Nicholson et al.[51] found that the expression of the epidermal growth factor receptor "is a highly significant marker of poor prognosis of breast cancer patients. . . ." Sainsbury et al.[52] reported that the epidermal growth factor receptor was a powerful predictor of recurrence in women with node-negative breast cancer. Indeed, Sainsbury went on to say that the epidermal growth factor receptor was a better single indicator (of prognosis) than node status. The immunohistochemistry and monoclonal antibodies necessary for this determination are not generally available at this time. If you are interested in learning more about the availability of this procedure, contact Adrian L. Harris, Cancer Research Unit, Royal Victoria Infirmary, Newcastle upon Tyme, U.K. NEI 4LP.

REFERENCES

1. Osborne CK, Receptors. In *Breast Diseases*. Harris, Hellman, Henderson, and Kinne, eds. Philadelphia: JB Lippincott, 1987, pp. 210–232.
2. Clark G, et al. Progesterone receptor as a prognostic factor in Stage II breast cancer. *N Eng J Med* 309:1343–1347, 1983.
3. Fisher B, Fisher ER, et al. Tumor nuclear grade, estrogen receptor, and progesterone receptor: their value alone or in combination as indicators of outcome following adjuvant therapy for breast cancer. *Breast Cancer Research and Treatment* 71:147–160, 1986.
4. Moran R, et al. Correlation of cell kinetics, hormone receptors, histopathology, and node status in human breast cancer. *Cancer* 54:1586–1590, 1984.
5. Chevallier B, et al. Prognostic value of estrogen and progesterone receptors in operable breast cancer. *Cancer* 62:2517–2524, 1988.
6. Sainsbury JR, et al. Epidermal growth factor receptor status as predictors of early recurrence of and death from breast cancer. *The Lancet* 1398–1402, June 20, 1987.
7. Osborne CK. *Oncology Viewpoints, Adjuvant Therapy in Node-Negative Breast Cancer.* L.P. Communications, Inc., 1988, p. 12.
8. Bloom HJK. Prognosis in breast cancer. *Br J Cancer* 4:259–288, 1950.

9. Parl FF, et al., A retrospective cohort study of histologic risk factors in breast cancer. *Cancer* 50:2410–2416, 1982.

10. Russo J, et al. Predictors of recurrence and survival of patients with breast cancer. *Am J Clin Pathol* 88:123—131,1987.

11. McDivitt RW, et al. A proposed classification of breast cancer based on kinetic information. *Cancer* 57:269–276, 1985.

12. Kuhns J G. Testimony in Linn County District Court, State of Iowa, *Deburkartre v. Louvar,* April 1985, Book 2.

13. Bloom HJK and Richarson WW. Histologic grading and prognosis in breast cancer. *Br J Cancer* 11:359–377, 1957.

14. Hanson DE. The histologic grading of neoplasms. *Arch Pathol Lab Med* 112:1091–1096, 1988.

15. Osborne CK. Prognostic factors. Oncology Viewpoints: Special Issue, Adjuvant Therapy in Node Negative Breast Cancer. Society of Clinical Oncologists. Page 12, LP Communications Inc., New York, N.Y., 1988.

16. Van Der Linden JC, Baak JP, Hermans J, and Meyer CJL. Prospective evaluation of prognostic value of morphometry in patients with primary breast cancer. *J Clin Pathol* 40:302–306, 1987.

17. Blamey RW, et al. A prognostic index in breast cancer—tested and confirmed. Abstract. *Breast Cancer Treatment and Research.* 4:335, 1984.

18. Haybittle JL, Blamey RW et al. A prognostic index in primary breast cancer. *British J Cancer* 45:361–366, 1982.

19. Todd JH et al. Confirmation of a prognostic index in primary breast cancer. *Br. J. Cancer* 56:489–492, 1987.

20. Heuser LS, et al. The association of pathologic and mammographic characteristics of primary breast cancer with "slow" and "fast" growth rates and with axillary lymph node metastases. *Cancer* 53:96–98, 1984.

21. Gilchrist KW quoted by Stern JW. Tumor necrosis can predict survival in breast cancer. *Oncology Times* 10(9): May 1988.

22. Blamey RW. et al. Factors influencing local recurrence after excision and radiotherapy for primary breast cancer. *Breast Cancer Research and Treatment* 12:(12) 117, 1988 (abstract).

23. Fisher E, et al. The pathology of invasive breast cancer. A

syllabus derived from the findings of the National Surgical Adjuvant Breast Project. (Protocol #4) *Cancer* 36:1–85, 1975.

24. Dressler LG, et al. DNA flow cytometry and prognostic factors in 1331 frozen breast cancer specimens. *Cancer* 61:420–427, 1988.

25. Clark G. DNA flow cytometry proving to be a useful tool by Carole Bullock. In *Oncology Times,* February 15, 198.

26. Auer G, et al. DNA content and survival in mammary carcinoma. *Anal Quant Cytol* 3:161–165, 1980.

27. Fallenius AG, et al. Predictive value of nuclear DNA content in breast cancer in relation to clinical and morphologic factors. A retrospective study of 227 consecutive cases. *Cancer* 62:521–530, 1988.

28. Hedley DW, et al. Method for analysis of cellular DNA content of paraffin embedded pathological material using flow cytometry. *J Histochem and Cytochem* 31:1333–1335,1983.

29. Clark GM, et al. Prediction of relapse or survival in patients with node-negative breast cancer by DNA flow cytometry. *N Eng J Med* 320(10):627–632, 1989.

30. Meyer JS. Cell kinetics of breast and breast tumors. In *Cancer of the Breast,* 3rd ed. Donegan and Spratt, eds. WB Saunders, 1988, p. 265.

31. Kornstein MJ. DNA flow cytometry in the prognosis of node negative women. Letter to the Editor. *N Engl J Med* 321:(7)473, August 17, 1989.

32. Clark GM and McQuire WL. Letter to the Editor . *N Engl J Med* 321:(7)474. August 17, 1989.

33. Hedley, David. Personal communication, September 9, 1987.

34. Beerman H et al. Letter to the Editor. *N Engl J Med.* 321:(7)473–474, August 17, 1989.

35. Ewers SB, Langstrom E, Baldetorp B, Killasnder D. Flow cytometric DNA analysis in primary breast carcinoma and clinicopathological correlations. *Cytometry* 5:408–419, 1984.

36. Harvey J, de Klerk N, Berryman I, Sterrett G, Byrne M, and Papandimitriou J. Nuclear DNA content and prognosis in human breast cancer: a static cytophotometric study. *Breast Cancer Res and Treat* 9:101–109, 1987.

37. Kallioniemi O-P, Blanco G, Alavaikko M et al. Improving

the prognostic value of DNA flow cytometry in breast cancer by combining DNA index and S-phase fraction: a proposed classification of DNA histograms in breast cancer. *Cancer* 62:2183–2190, 1988.

38. Retsky MW, et al. Prospective computerized simulation of breast cancer: a comparison of computer predictions with nine sets of biological and clinical data. *Cancer Research* 47:4982–4987, 1987.
39. Retsky MW. Personal communication, June 30, 1989.
40. Baack JP, et al. The value of morphometry to classic prognosticators in breast cancer. *Cancer* 56:374–382, 1985.
41. Maehle BO, et al. Mean nuclear area and histologic grade of axillary node tumors in breast cancer. *Br J Cancer* 46:95–100, 1982.
42. McDivitt RW, et al. Tumors of the breast. In *Atlas of Tumor Pathology*, 2nd Series, fascicle number 2. Bethesda, MD: Armed Forces Institute of Pathology, 1967, p. 86.
43. Rosen PP. The pathology of breast carcinoma. In *Breast Diseases*, Harris, Hellman, Henderson, and Kinne, eds. JB Lippincott, 1987, p. 156.
44. Fox AS. On the diagnosis and treatment of breast cancer. *JAMA* 241:489–494, 1979.
45. Hellman S. The primary treatment of breast cancer, concluding remarks. In *Breast Diseases*. Harris, Hellman, Henderson, and Kinne, eds. JB Lippincott, 1987, p. 354.
46. Henderson JC. Prognostic factors. Oncology Viewpoints, Special Issue, Adjuvant Therapy in Node Negative Breast Cancer. Society of Clinical Oncology. LP Communications Inc. New York, NY 1988, p. 14.
47. Kuhajda FP, Piantadosi S, and Pasternack, GR. Haptoglobin-related protein (Hpr) epitopes in breast cancer as a predictor of recurrence of the disease. *N Engl J Med* 321(10):636–641. 1989.
48. Weiss R. Marker predicts breast cancer recurrence. *Science News* 136:(11)163, September 9, 1989.
49. Clark M and McQuire W L. New biologic prognostic factors in breast cancer. *Oncology* 3:(5)49–64 May 1989.
50. Tandon A, Clark G, and Ullrich A et al. Overexpression of the HER2/neu oncogene predicts relapse and survival in

stage II human breast cancer. *Proc Am Soc Clin Oncol* 7:14, 1988.

51. Nicholson et al. Expression of epidermal growth factor receptors associated with lack of response to endocrine therapy in recurrent breast cancer. *The Lancet* 1 (8631): 182–185.

52. Sainsbury J, Richard C et al. Epidermal growth-factor receptor status as predictor of early recurrence of and death from breast cancer. *The Lancet* 1398-1402, June 20, 1987.

GLOSSARY

ADENOSIS An overgrowth of glandular tissue, usually benign.

ANAPLASTIC Immature, undifferentiated; an aggressive and rapidly growing cancer.

ANEUPLOID A cancer cell with an abnormal amount of DNA, usually increased in amount. Aneuploid breast cancers have a higher rate of treatment failure than diploid breast cancers.

ATYPIA The term *epithelial hyperplasia* with *atypia* suggests that some of the hyperplastic cells have the appearance of malignant cells, but careful examination has revealed no evidence of invasion. These lesions are, therefore, considered to be premalignant. Many of these lesions will become malignant.

BIAS, LEAD TIME Routine screening examinations often detect cancers earlier in their life cycle. Some of these women will live a year or two longer and will still die of breast cancer. This falsely improves the survival rate.

BIAS, LENGTH Rapidly growing cancers frequently surface between screening examinations. Slow-growing cancers, on the other hand, are more often detected during routine screening examinations. Since these tumors have a better survival rate, this falsely improves the survival rate.

BIAS, SELCTION Physicians unconsciously tend to eliminate patients with unfavorable cancers.

BIOLOGIC PREDETERMINATION The nature of the damage to the DNA of a cancer cell at the moment of its inception, or early in its life cycle, determines the future behavior of the tumor. This frequently occurs long before it is possible to detect the cancer by any presently available diagnostic modality.

CAMOUFLAGED TUMOR A tumor whose presence within the the breast is hidden or masked from the clinician's palpating fingers and/or the X-ray beam because the density of the breast and tumor are similar or the tumor contains no calcifications. Some tumors, because of their peculiar pattern of invasion, are more likely to become camouflaged.

CAPILLARY A small blood vessel that connects a terminal artery to the venous collecting system of veins.

CARCINOGEN Any cancer-producing substance.

CHROMOSOME A long coiled and twisted strand of DNA containing genetic information. There are 46 chromosomes in all human cells except the ovum and sperm which contain 23.

CRITICAL SIZE The size at which a tumor first acquires the ability to spread systemically, often soon after the tumor becomes vascularized.

CYTOMETRY See *flow cytometry*.

DESMOPLASIA An overgrowth of fibrous tissue.

DIAMETER, DOUBLING When a breast cancer undergoes three net cell generations, there is an eightfold increase in mass (2–4–8). An eightfold increase in mass results in a doubling of the diameter of the tumor.

DIPLOID A cell that has two sets of chromosomes as are normally found in the nuclei of all human cells. Breast cancer cells with diploid DNA tend to have a better prognosis than aneuploid cancer cells. The DNA index of a diploid tumor is 1.0.

    HYPODIPLOID DNA content slightly less than normal (diploid), these tumors are said to have a poor prognosis. The DNA index of these tumors would be less than 1.0.

    HYPERDIPLOID DNA content slightly greater than normal but less than fourfold (tetraploid). The DNA index would be slightly above 1.0.

DISEASE-FREE INTERVAL The length of time between the surgical removal of a breast cancer and the first evidence of recurrence of the tumor.

DNA Deoxyribonucleic acid. An acid consisting of four nucleic acids (adenine, guanine, cytosine, and thymine) which are strung together like beads on a long strand of tissue composed of a carbohydrate and a protein. The four nucleic acids form the four-letter alphabet (A-G-C-T) of the genetic code. All human cells contain DNA in their nuclei.

DNA FLOW CYTOMETRY See *flow cytometry.*

DNA INDEX Refers to the amount of DNA in a breast cancer cell. Normal breast cells have a DNA index of 1.0. Cancer cells with a DNA of greater than 1.0 have a greater than normal amount of DNA in their nuclei. Those with a DNA index of less than 1.0 have a less than normal amount of DNA in their nuclei. The DNA index correlates with the survival rate.

DOUBLING TIME The time required for a tumor to double the number of cancer cells within the tumor. Three net cell doublings of a tumor results in an eightfold increase in mass and a doubling of the diameter of the tumor.

DYSPLASIA An abnormal overgrowth of benign tissue, sometimes premalignant.

EMBOLUS A tumor embolus is a small cluster of cancer cells which has become detached from a cancer and is carried away by the flow of blood or lymph to a distant location.

ENZYME A protein capable of accelerating a chemical reaction, usually a specific chemical reaction.

ESTROGEN AND PROGESTERONE RECEPTOR Normal breast cells and some breast cancer cells contain special proteins called receptors. These receptors attach to estrogen and progesterone in the nucleus of the cell where they initiate certain vital functions. The presence of the estrogen receptor (ER) and the progesterone receptor (PgR) in the cytoplasm of a tumor is a sign of maturity, and tumors that are ER + /PgR + grow more slowly and have a better survival rate than ER – / PgR – tumors. Hormone receptors are reported as fematomoles per milligram of cytosol protein. Tumors with less than 3 to 9 f/mols per milligram of cytosol protein are usually considered to be negative. (The exact cutoff varies with different laboratories.) *Femto* is a Danish word for 15, and in this case means 10^{-15} or one-quadrillionth of a mole. A mole (*mol*) is an abbreviation for molecular weight.

FEMTO A Danish word that means 15. See *estrogen and progesterone receptors.*

FIBROCYTE OR FIBROBLAST A connective tissue cell.

FLOW CYTOMETRY A suspension of free tumor nuclei is created by treating a tumor mechanically and/or with enzymes. The DNA within the tumor nuclei is stained with a dye that becomes fluorescent when struck with a beam of a laser light. The suspension of tumor nuclei is then forced through the cytometer under pressure in such a fashion that the cell suspension is broken into a fine stream of droplets, each containing a single tumor nuclei. As the tumor nuclei passes through the beam of laser light, a computer records the amount of DNA in each nucleus by measuring the degree of fluorescence of each nucleus. Flow cytometry provides us with two important pieces of information:

1. It gives us an accurate measurement of the percentage of tumor cells that are in the synthetic S-phase fraction of cell division, that is, the number of cells that are in the process of doubling their DNA prior to cell division.

2. It measures the DNA content of each tumor nucleus. If the amount of DNA in the tumor cells is normal or near normal, the tumor is said to be diploid and seems to have a better prognosis. If the amount of DNA is increased or decreased, the tumor is said to be aneuploid. Aneuploid tumors have a poorer prognosis than diploid tumors. The greater the distortion of the DNA, the more aggressive the breast cancer.

GENE A small segment of DNA that carries a specific message.

GRANULOCYTE A white blood cell which usually fights infection.

HETEROGENEOUS Complosed of dissimilar parts.

HISTOLOGY The microscopic anatomy of a tissue.

HYPERDIPLOID See *diploid.*

HYPODIPLOID See *diploid.*

HYPERPLASIA An abnormal overgrowth of a tissue, usually benign.

HYPERTETRAPLOID See *tetraploid.*

INTERVAL TUMOR A breast cancer that surfaces within 12 months of a negative screening examination.

KARYORRHEXIS The rupture of a cell nucleus with dispersion of the chromatin from the cell nucleus.

LEAD TIME BIAS See *bias.*

LENGTH BIAS See *bias.*

MACROPHAGE A large white cell that can ingest necrotic tissue, debris, and kill bacteria.

MATRIX The substance that binds together the various structures and molecules within a cell.

METASTASIS The spread of a cell or a cluster of cancer cells to distant organs via the blood or lymph.

MITOTIC INDEX The number of mitotic figures (dividing cells) in 10 high power fields of an ordinary light microscope.

MITOSIS The act of cell division.

MOL An abbreviation for mole or molecular weight.

MOLE An abbreviation for molecular weight.

MUTATION From the Latin, *to change.* This refers to a change in the genetic message brought about by an abnormal cell division.

MYOFIBROBLAST A contractile fibroblast.

NECROSIS The death of tissue or cells.

NUCLEAR MORPHOMETRY An inexpensive and seldom used procedure. A photomicrograph is greatly enlarged and projected onto a special screen marked with vertical and horizontal lines so placed that the nuclear diameter and area can be readily measured and recorded in um^2. (um^2 means square microns or 1/1,000 of a millimeter.) The mitotic index can also be easily measured by this technique. The mean nuclear area, mean nuclear diameter, and mitotic index all correlate well with prognosis.

ONCOGENE A unit of genetic information that specifies a protein that controls mitosis (cell division). The term *specifies* means that this gene supplies the instructions to the cell that enable it to manufacture a protein capable of controlling and modulating cell division.

OSMOSIS The diffusion of fluids and small particles through membranes or porous partitions.

PLOIDY A Greek word meaning *a fold.* Therefore, ploidy refers to the gross configuration of the DNA. The greater the increase in the DNA beyond the normal amount, the more aggressive the cancer.

PRETHRESHOLD SIZE See *threshold size.*

PROGESTERONE RECEPTOR A protein complex that attaches to progesterone in the nucleus of the cell. See also *estrogen* *receptor.* Some say the progesterone receptor also transports progesterone to the nucleus.

PROLIFERATION RATE The growth rate of a cancer, commonly measured by the mitotic index, the thymidine labeling index, or the S-phase fraction determined by flow cytometry. Tumors with a high proliferation rate are growing more rapidly than the average breast cancer, are more aggressive, and have a high rate of treatment failure.

PROTO-ONCOGENE A unit of genetic information that controls and modulates normal mitosis (cell division). That is, the proto-oncogene supplies the cell with the information necessary to manufacture a protein which has the ability to control and modulate normal cell division. When the proto-oncogene is damaged by a carcinogen, it programs the cell to manufacture an abnormal protein which instructs the cell to grow continuously. Thus a cancer has developed. These damaged proto-oncogenes are then called oncogenes (Janet Rowley, quoted by Ruth SoRelle in *Oncology Times,* January 15, 1988, p. 2). See also *Oncogene.*

PYKNOSIS The shrunken nucleus of a degenerating cell.

R1–R2 INTERVAL The interval between the detection of the first metastasis and the second metastasis. A short R1-R2 interval suggests a rapid proliferation rate.

SELECTION BIAS See *bias.*

SHEDDING The escape of cancer cells or small clusters of cancer cells into the blood or lymph.

SLIDING THRESHOLD SIZE See *threshold size.*

S-PHASE FRACTION Cancer cells whose DNA is in the synthesis phase (in the process of doubling of their DNA prior to cell division) are said to be in the S-phase. The S-phase is the first phase of cell division. Determining the numbers of cells in the S-phase is one of the most accurate methods for measuring the proliferation rate of a breast cancer.

STAGE CREEP Over the years the improvements in our diagnostic tests have made it possible to diagnose recurrent breast cancer at a much earlier stage. These patients are then shifted to the next higher stage with more serious disease. This falsely improves the survival since the overall survival rate remains the same.

STROMA The supporting tissue framework of an organ such as the breast; primarily connective tissue (sometimes called fibrous tissue).

TETRAPLOID Normal cells have diploid (twofold) DNA content. Some tumor cells have double the amount of normal DNA and are therefore called tetraploid (fourfold). The DNA index of a tetraploid tumor cell would be 2.0.

> **HYPERTETRAPLOID** Tumor cells that contain more than double the amount of normal DNA (tetraploid). The DNA index of the hypertetraploid would be greater than 2.0.

THRESHOLD SIZE The smallest size at which it is possible to detect a breast cancer. We speak of the threshold size by palpation and the threshold size by mammography.

> **PRETHRESHOLD SIZE** A tumor that is too small to be detected by the particular examination under discussion.

> **SLIDING THRESHOLD SIZE** There is an enormous variation in the threshold size which is secondary to variations in the density and consistency of the breast and/or the tumor.

THYMIDINE LABELING INDEX (TLI) One of the most accurate measurements of the proliferation rate of breast cancer. It is performed as follows:

1. The amino acid thymine is unique in that it is found only in DNA.

2. However, thymine cannot enter the cell nucleus unless it is attached to a sugar.

3. Therefore, a sugar is attached to thymine and becomes thymidine.

4. Thymidine is tagged with a radioactive tracer (H3) and placed upon a thin slice of fresh tumor tissue. The thin slice of fresh tumor tissue, covered with the radioactive thymidine, is then incubated for several hours so that the tumor cells that are in the process of cell division will incorporate the radioactive thymidine into the DNA of their nuclei.

5. The tissue is removed from the incubator and flooded with water to wash away the radioactive thymidine that was not taken up and and incorporated into the DNA during the period of incubation.

6. The thin slice of tumor tissue is then covered with pho-

tographic emulsion and placed in a dark container for several days. During this time the radioactive material in the newly formed DNA will develop the photographic emulsion overlying the nuclei containing radioactive DNA.

7. The number of nuclei containing tiny specs of silver are then counted, and from this, the percentage of cells in the process of cell division can be determined.

The thymidine labeling index (TLI) is seldom used in clinical practice because it requires fresh tumor tissue and is quite expensive. However, it is one of the most accurate ways to measure the proliferation rate of breast cancer. It serves as a standard against which we can compare the value of the various parameters for determing the prognosis of breast cancer. For example, tumors with a poor nuclear grade also have a high TLI. This tells us that tumors with a poor nuclear grade have a high proliferation and therefore have a high risk of developing recurrence of their cancer.

TUMOR, DIAMETER Three net cell generations (doublings) produces an eightfold increase in mass. When the mass of a tumor increases eight times, the diameter of the tumor will double.

VASCULARIZATION The process of developing a blood supply.

INDEX

Aneuploid breast cancers, 114–115, 171
Axillary lymph node metastases
  myths about, 100
  risk factors and, 76–78

Bias
  mass screening studies and, 36–37
  retrospective studies with, 35–36
Biologic Predetermination, 3–7
Breast cancer
  biologic predetermination for, 3–7
  common myths about, 99–107
  malignant potential of, 71–73, 155–180
  natural history of, 9–14
  treatment of, *see* Treatment of breast cancer

Cancer cells
  biologic predetermination and, 3–7
  diagnosis and tumor density and, 24–25
  natural history of breast cancer and, 9–10
  shedding of, 52–55
Cell doubling time, 10–14
Clinical studies, common sources of error in, 35–40
Computer programs, 145, 174
Critical size in diagnosis, 17–18
Cross-examination, and expert witnesses, 43–44

Cure
  biologic predetermination and, 5
  challenging expert witness on, 129–131
  time of diagnosis and, 101–102
Cystic mastitis, chronic, 24

Defense, 133–149
  assembling medical facts for, 69–84
  challenges to medical data presented by, 109–117
  checklist for pathologist and, 72–73
  checklist for radiologist in, 80–81
  doubling time and, 85–94, 147–148
  expert witness for, 43
  focus on overall problem in, 69–71
  malignant potential of breast cancer and, 71–73
  palpation of breast and, 82–84
  risk factors and, 73–79
  sliding threshold size and, 95–98
Density of breast tissue, and diagnosis, 23–24, 32–33, 82
Density of tumor, and diagnosis, 24–25
Diagnosis, 15–20
  average size of breast tumor at, 13–14
  breast consistency and, 24
  breast density and, 23–24
  breast size and, 24
  camouflaged tumor and, 23–29
  common myths about, 99–102
  critical size and, 17–18
  disagreements over spread and, 18–19

Diagnosis (*cont'd*)
  early, 15–16, 41–42, 119–127, 134–138
  interval tumor and, 31–34
  lateness of, 121–123
  retrospective studies and, 35
  staging systems and, 102–106
  survival rate and delay in, 19–20
  threshold size and, 17
  tumor density and, 24–25
Diploid breast cancers, 114, 170–171
DNA index, 172
Doubling time
  calculating, 87–89
  cells and, 10–14, 51–52, 61–67
  defense arguments with, 85–94,
    147–148
  metastasis and, 91–92, 116–117
  size of tumor and, 90–91
Duct cell carcinoma, infiltrating, 26–27

Early diagnosis, 15–16, 41–42, 119–127,
  134–138
Estrogen receptor (ER), 73–74, 110–111,
  120, 145, 155–159
Expert witnesses
  challenging, 129–131
  selecting, 43–44

Flow cytometry, 75–76, 113–115, 116,
  121, 169–174

Genetic predetermination to breast
  cancer, 3–7
Grading of tumor cells, 112, 159–160,
  164–165
Growth factors, 179–180
Growth of breast tumor
  challenges to medical data on, 115–117
  DNA status and, 55–59
  early diagnosis and, 41–42
  educating jury about, 45–46
  histologic features and, 159–166
  interval tumors and, 33
  natural history and, 10–14
  posterboard presentation on, 50–51
  presenting defense data on, 70–71

Growth of breast tumor (*cont'd*)
  survival rate and, 120–121
  threshold size and, 147

Haptoglobin-related protein (Hpr),
  178–179
Histologic features of breast cancer,
  175–177
  growth rate and, 159–166
  risk factors and, 74–75
Historical perspective on breast cancer
  treatment, 1–2
Hormone receptors, and risk factors,
  73–74, 110–111, 120

Infiltrating duct cell carcinoma, 26–27
Infiltrating lobular carcinoma, 25–26
Interval tumor, 31–34, 138–141
  doubling and, 61–67
  presenting defense data on, 70–71
Intraductal carcinoma, 27

Jury
  assembling medical facts for defense
    and, 69–84
  common myths about breast cancer
    and, 99–107
  cross-examination of expert
    witnesses and, 43–44
  education of, 45–67
  opening statement to, 46
  posterboard presentation to, 47–66
  selecting members of, 46
  sliding threshold defense and, 98

Lobular carcinoma, infiltrating, 25–26
Lymph node metastases
  risk factors and, 76–78
  tumor grading and, 165–166

Malignant potential of breast cancer,
  71–73, 155–180

Mammography
  camouflaged tumor on, 23–29
  clinical data errors and, 36–37
  interval tumor and, 31–34
  limitations of, 37–40
  medullary carcinoma on, 27
  risk factors and, 79–82
  sliding threshold defense and, 96–97
  threshold size with, 141–142
  technical problems with, 37–40
Mastectomy, 2
Medullary carcinoma, 27–28
Metastases
  biologic predetermination and, 6
  common myths about, 100–101
  critical size in diagnosis and, 17–18
  disagreements about rate of, 18–19
  doubling and, 91–92, 116–117
  early diagnosis and, 41–42
  historical perspective on, 1–2
  interval tumor and, 138–139
  posterboard presentation on, 47–49
  risk factors and, 76–78
Mitotic index, 111–112, 161–164
Mortality
  biologic predetermination and, 5–6
  early diagnosis and, 15–16

Natural history of breast cancer, 9–14
Nuclear morphometry, 76, 174–175

Oncogenes, 179
Opening statement, 46

Palpation, 82–84, 96–97, 142–145
Parenchymal patterns, 81–82
Pathologists, 144
  checklist for, 72–73
  cross-examination of, 43–44
  malignancy of breast cancer and, 71–72
Plaintiff, expert witness for, 43–44
Posterboard presentation
  examples of, 47–67
  preparing, 47
Progesterone receptor (PgR), 73–74,
    110–111, 120, 145, 155–159

Radiologist, checklist for, 80–81
Recurrence of tumor, as risk factor, 79
Retrospective studies, limitation of, 35–36
Risk factors, 145
  evaluating, 73–79, 147
  listing, 73
  microscopic, 167–169
  predictive value of, 113, 166–167

Screening programs
  clinical data errors and, 36–37
  diagnosis and survival rates and, 16–18
  frequency of, 123–127
  interval tumor and, 31–33
Size of breast, and diagnosis, 24
Size of tumor
  common myths about, 99
  doubling and, 90–91
  growth rate and, 147
  lymph node status and, 165–166
  mammography for, 141–142
  palpation and, 142–145
  risk factors and, 78–79
  sliding threshold defense and, 95–98
Sliding threshold, 60, 95–98
Staging systems, 102–106
Survival rates
  delay in diagnosis and, 19–20
  early diagnosis and, 15–16, 119–127
  mitotic index and, 111–112
  screening programs and diagnosis
    and, 16–18

Threshold size in diagnosis, 17, 60–61,
    141–142, 147
T-N-M staging system, 102–106, 144
Treatment of breast cancer
  historical perspective on, 1–2

Vascularization of breast tumor, 12, 49–50

Witnesses
  challenging, 129–131
  selecting, 43–44
Wolfe's parenchymal patterns, 81–82